Being Critically Reflective

Pete
Connolly

(2014 — Edition)

Practice Theory in Context series
Series Editor: Jan Fook

Change is rife in welfare organisations but expectations for sound and effective practice continue to rise. More than ever, professionals need to be able to remake ideas and principles for relevance in a range of different circumstances as well as transfer learning from one context to the next.

This new series focuses on approaches to practice that are common and prevalent in health and social care settings. Each book succinctly explains the theoretical principles of its approach and shows exactly how these ideas can be applied skilfully in the pressurised world of day-to-day practice.

Pitched at a level suitable for students on introductory courses, the books are holistic in ethos, also considering organisational and policy contexts, working with colleagues, ethics and values, self-care and professional development. As such, these texts are ideal too as theory refreshers for early and later career practitioners.

Published

Laura Beres
The Narrative Practitioner

Fiona Gardner
Being Critically Reflective

Being Critically Reflective

Engaging in Holistic Practice

Fiona Gardner

palgrave
macmillan

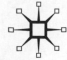

© Fiona Gardner 2014

All rights reserved. No reproduction, copy or transmission of this
publication may be made without written permission.

No portion of this publication may be reproduced, copied or transmitted
save with written permission or in accordance with the provisions of the
Copyright, Designs and Patents Act 1988, or under the terms of any licence
permitting limited copying issued by the Copyright Licensing Agency,
Saffron House, 6-10 Kirby Street, London EC1N 8TS.

Any person who does any unauthorized act in relation to this publication
may be liable to criminal prosecution and civil claims for damages.

The author has asserted her right to be identified as the author of this
work in accordance with the Copyright, Designs and Patents Act 1988.

First published 2014 by
PALGRAVE MACMILLAN

Palgrave Macmillan in the UK is an imprint of Macmillan Publishers Limited,
registered in England, company number 785998, of Houndmills, Basingstoke,
Hampshire RG21 6XS.

Palgrave Macmillan in the US is a division of St Martin's Press LLC,
175 Fifth Avenue, New York, NY 10010.

Palgrave Macmillan is the global academic imprint of the above companies
and has companies and representatives throughout the world.

Palgrave® and Macmillan® are registered trademarks in the United States,
the United Kingdom, Europe and other countries

ISBN: 978–1–137–27667–4

This book is printed on paper suitable for recycling and made from fully
managed and sustained forest sources. Logging, pulping and manufacturing
processes are expected to conform to the environmental regulations of the
country of origin.

A catalogue record for this book is available from the British Library.

A catalog record for this book is available from the Library of Congress.

Typeset by Cambrian Typesetters, Camberley, Surrey

Printed in China

Contents

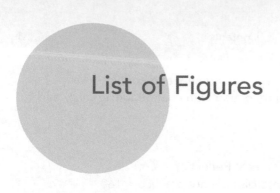

List of Figures

Acknowledgements

With thanks to all those who have been part of the journey of being critically reflective and particularly to Drew.

Introduction

Those who work in health, education and social care are faced with increasing challenges in the complexity of their practice and the context in which they operate. Critical reflection provides a theoretical approach to help understand these challenges as well as a process for engaging constructively with the dilemmas and issues that inevitably arise in professional practice. Essentially, critical reflection encourages practitioners to identify the underlying assumptions and values that influence their practice and to consider how they can act in line with their preferred assumptions and values. Being able to name these most deeply held values reminds practitioners of the underlying or fundamental reasons for their participation in this kind of practice. This, in itself, can be restoring and energizing as well as challenging and sometimes even painful. The sense of working from fundamental values reinforces the integrity inherent for practitioners in their practice or what they might name as the meaningful or spiritual dimension. Practitioners have affirmed that a critically reflective approach frequently grounded and centred them, taking them to a place where they were reminded of their sense of altruism and hope about their work. While this did not necessarily resolve the dilemmas of practice, it frequently enabled practitioners to engage more actively with them, seeing new perspectives and possibilities for change either for themselves or in their practice. Where change was not possible externally, practitioners suggest they generally became more able to manage living with the uncertainties and complexities of practice. This was both enabling and restoring, and paradoxically encouraged them to take greater care of themselves, partly so that they could be more effective practitioners.

The need for such a critically reflective approach is imperative in an environment of rapid social and economic change where organizations and practitioners are experiencing greater demands in a context of fewer resources; what Baker (2013, p. 126) in the United Kingdom refers to as the 'current stringent and streamlined climate'. Uncertainty and the rate of change are increasing and these contribute to higher levels of conflict and ethical challenges both in organizations and in society generally. The 'domination of practice by procedures and bureaucracy' combined with greater service user complexity increases anxiety for practitioners (Ruch, 2005, p. 112). Given that practice usually happens within an organizational context and always within a societal context, a critically reflective approach enables practitioners to stand back from the immediate to consider the implications of the broader context and the connections to the underlying values of practice (Oliver and Keeping, 2010).

Funding pressures can also add weight to expectations of increased 'interprofessional' practice both within and between organizations. Such practice focuses on what tasks can be shared across professional disciplines to encourage collaborative practices. From a service-user perspective this can have advantages of more accessible and better coordinated service delivery. However, interprofessional practice can be confronting for practitioners who value their distinct professional identity and who struggle with differences in philosophy and language from other professions. The focus on efficiencies can also mean pressure to reduce practice to common competencies or measurable work tasks without the more nuanced intuitive judgements and processes of a holistic approach to professional practice (Sturgeon, 2010).

Paradoxically, increased financial stringency means practitioners often feel less able to access critical reflection at a time when they need it more. Practitioners exhausted by increasing workloads and pressures of accountability for time and resources, find it almost impossible to see how they can create time for reflection. Reflective processes where the focus is on learning from what hasn't gone well can also feel dangerous in periods of redundancies and cuts. Organizations that have previously supported and possibly funded formal critical reflection processes may no longer see these as a priority. This book explores how practitioners can creatively generate their own structures or processes to support being critically reflective when their organizational context does not allow for or encourage this. Using critical reflection processes can enable practitioners to see the influence of the context more clearly rather than taking responsibility for what is beyond their capacity to change individually. Starting from a particular experience, practitioners can put into perspective what is happening in the broader context and its influence on them as well as identifying how their reaction to it is influenced by their own particular history and sense of self. From my own experience, I know that to share an issue in critical reflection can save time and energy, clarifying the influence of context, my reactions and my perspectives relatively quickly. Seeing the issue more clearly means I can then decide whether to do something differently, or whether I simply need to let it go. Either way, it has less power for sapping my energy.

It is clear that the expectation across professional disciplines is that some form of reflective practice or critical reflection will be part of student education and of professional practice. What is meant by this varies considerably with some writers/practitioners using critical reflection, reflective practice and reflexivity interchangeably and others attributing different meanings to the same language. These differences will be explored in the first chapter. Critical reflection, as used in this book, is about the capacity to be reflective, to make explicit the connections between values and assumptions underlying emotions, thoughts and reactions. The critical aspect relates to connecting these assumptions and values to the broader social context in a way that encourages action and particularly socially just action.

Critical reflection, as defined here, is practiced by practitioners across a wide range of health, education and social care settings in many countries (Fook and Gardner, 2013). The theory and process provides a common language for practitioners across many disciplines to explore their practice and how to work together more effectively. Critical reflection is used by managers, those supervising students and staff, those researching and evaluating practice as well as practitioners and students. People using critical reflection come from an increasingly diverse range of areas of practice including mental health, counselling, palliative care, rehabilitation, acute care, community development, youth services, family and children's services and aged care. While the experience of critical reflection may be influenced by the particular field of practice and the organizational context, it is clear from practitioners that the theory and processes are universally helpful (Fook and Gardner, 2013).

The title of this book is significant: *being* critically reflective is about an attitude to practice as well as the *doing* of critical reflection. Ideally, critical reflection permeates professional practice, influencing the stance taken to organizational life in general as well as to specific professional activities. The danger of some training about critical reflection is that it becomes solely a distinct activity that takes place in a formal forum such as supervision or in response to a particular event. In this book, I am suggesting that it is more helpful to generate an attitude or underlying perspective that is critically reflective. You could also argue that being critically reflective is an attitude to life in general, the desire to approach all aspects of life with the same spirit of enquiry; seeking to understand more deeply the underlying values and reactions to the everyday as well as to professional practice. Certainly, there are times when practitioners use critical reflection to make links between what is happening in their professional practice and in their personal lives. However, this book will focus primarily on using critical reflection in professional practice. As one practitioner wrote:

What stands out for me … using critical reflection is the inherent value of this process, journey, in supporting me in my everyday moments, challenges and relationships. Specifically, how an experience, in reflection, can beg my attention, interrupt my focus and keep bugging me until I reflect on its message, meaning, asking: 'what is this story I'm digesting, retelling, authoring about?' It's exhausting, magical, perplexing, freeing, inflating, deflating, true, rubbish, personal, public and funny. Maybe I'm all of these moods and contexts in the critical reflection process, so that it becomes not a thing that I 'do' but a way to 'be'. (Hanlon, 2009)

I have come to suggest this way of thinking about critical reflection as a result of my own experience with it and it fits with a critically reflective approach for me to be explicit about this, to name 'where I am coming from'. My own professional background is social work and when I started practicing as a social worker, the expectation to be reflective was more implicit than explicit. Social workers were expected to be aware of their own values and attitudes and how these might influence their practice, particularly in relation to work with individuals and families. This awareness was influenced by the greater emphasis on the psychodynamic approach prevalent at the time, which has also continued to influence my practice. I could certainly see in both my own practice and when I became a supervisor in the practice of others the need for constant self-awareness about how easily reactions are influenced by our own experience and values. I was also conscious, and social work training helped with this, of how community values and social expectations influenced me and those I worked with, both colleagues and service users. Having a variety of social work roles in government organizations, voluntary agencies and community-based settings reinforced my understanding of how the organizational context also impacted professional practice. Each of these settings came with its own set of understandings, assumptions and values both at informal and formal levels.

When I started teaching social work students in the mid-1990s, I was conscious that in teaching we needed to articulate these issues very clearly. We expected students to reflect on the assumptions, values and experiences that had influenced them to do social work, for example, but also how these experiences and values might influence them as workers. While there was significant agreement about the need for this aspect of professional training to be well developed, there were differences about how best to teach and particularly how to assess it. I was conscious too that for some of the students this was a particularly challenging area. For some, this was a new way of thinking about their approach to practice, something quite unexpected in what they had seen as a primarily academic course. For others the challenge was revealing what they saw as personal information that they were unsure would be accepted by their fellow students. This meant articulating more clearly the links between the personal and professional, the need for awareness of values and attitudes, the desirability of constant reflection.

This was reinforced for me by being seconded to the Centre for Professional Development coordinated by Jan Fook in the early 2000s. Jan had already been developing a framework for critical reflection in teaching social work students and had started to use critical reflection in workshops with professionals. The Centre had funding for three years supported by La Trobe University and the State Government Department of Human Services in Victoria, Australia. Over the next four years we ran a significant number of workshops for professionals from primarily health and welfare disciplines but also from education and law. In the process we refined the two stage model of critical reflection and this is described in detail in Fook and Gardner (2007). We also edited a book with Sue White (White, Fook and Gardner, 2006) where contributors explored frameworks for understanding critical reflection and how critical reflection was used in professional learning, research and education. More recently we edited a book where practitioners have identified how they used or adapted the two stage model of critical reflection in their practice as well as in research and education (Fook and Gardner, 2013).

While I was at the Centre, I began to see that part of what was important to many practitioners about critical reflection was the clearer identification of what their practice meant to them. The values that were fundamental emerged in the course of critically reflecting about a particular experience. As these values emerged, practitioners were restored to a place of meaning and integrity. They were able to clarify what really mattered to them in terms of their practice, the values from which they wanted to operate. It became clearer for these practitioners where their values were in conflict with what they had felt or done. This sense of returning to what matters resonated for me with my interest in the spiritual, which can also be seen in terms of what matters, what gives meaning. As a result of this, I ran some workshops from the Centre called 'Spirituality and Work'. These workshops were based on the theory and practice of critical reflection but in a more implicit way. The practitioners attending the spirituality workshops were primarily interested in engaging with issues of how to include spirituality in practice.

Soon after this, I returned to the Department of Social Work and Social Policy (at La Trobe University, based in Bendigo) and became involved in two research projects. One of these, the Pastoral Care Networks Project (Gardner and Nolan, 2009) provided training for practitioners and volunteers involved in palliative care and related services. The focus of the training was spirituality/pastoral care and the training, like the Spirituality and Work workshops, was based on the theory and practice of critical reflection being implicit rather than explicit. The training was primarily experiential, encouraging participants to use specific experiences to explore their own sense of the spiritual, how this might vary from other people and how this might influence their practice. The training also provided input about the social and historical context of palliative care: how this has and continues to influence how we care for those who are dying, attitudes to religion and spirituality and the role of community. The second project, Health Promoting Palliative Care, (Gardner, Rumbold and Salau, 2009) used critical reflection in the evaluation of the Project and in running workshops on how to engage with issues of death and dying in local communities. This led to writing more specifically about 'critical spirituality' (Gardner, 2011).

At the same time, I continued to run critical reflection workshops and to facilitate critical reflection supervision groups, particularly in health settings and to see some people for individual supervision, again using critical reflection. This range of experiences prompted me to think about the differences between people who chose to use critical reflection from time to time, in a group or an individual supervision, as opposed to those who seem to 'adopt' critical reflection. For this second group of people critical reflection seemed to become an integral part of their practice rather than something they 'did'. Having this attitude to critical reflection or rather than having this critically reflecting attitude to their practice meant that these practitioners tended to approach all of their practice from this perspective. There were clearly advantages in this for them. They were able to ask critically reflective questions during short encounters in passageways easily, to question their own actions or thoughts in the process of their work, rather than to question separate experiences in retrospect. This made me consider the value of encouraging practitioners to *be* critically reflective rather than only participating in specific critical reflection activities. This is not to say that such practitioners did not also find value in specific critical reflection activities such as individual or group supervision. They continued to appreciate how these reinforced their critically reflective attitude. They also acknowledged that there remained times when they needed another person's perspective or questions, a formal critically reflective process when they were engaged with somebody else in order to disentangle their feelings, thoughts and assumptions.

This fits with my own experience of critical reflection. When I think about how engaged I have been with critically reflective processes, my sense is that this is an integral part of how I approach my practice. However, I can still find myself needing the formality of a critical reflection interaction with someone who is aware of the process, can ask appropriate questions and enable me to unearth the feelings, thoughts, assumptions and values that are influencing my reactions in a particular context. I now meet regularly with a colleague for mutual critical reflection sessions.

Much has been written about critical reflection and reflective practice in recent years, for particular disciplines such as nursing and social work and across disciplines. What then is distinctive about this book?

First, this book advocates *being* critically reflective as an attitude of mind as well as *doing* critical reflection. I am not suggesting a dichotomy here of *being* critically reflective *versus doing*; as I've suggested from my own and others experience, the aim is to combine both. It is probably more accurate to acknowledge that people will reflect in different ways at different times with strands of being and doing critical reflection intertwining over time at varying levels. People also differ in their preferences for how they reflect and when, and what suits their particular personalities and personal and professional histories (Hickson, 2013). For some people being critically reflective comes easily: some participants in workshops will say, this fits with how I am, I can see that I've always been actively reflective this helps me name and focus this, be more articulate about it. For others, critical reflection is quite different from their normal way of being, a typical comment might be this feels quite alien to me, I'm much more a task-oriented person, doing comes more naturally than reflecting on it.

However, there are clearly advantages in seeking to cultivate an attitude of *being* critical reflective rather than seeing this as purely a monthly event that happens at something like a supervision session. The implication is that if you are being critically reflective as a worker this will influence your practice with all those you work with – service users, communities as well as colleagues. Feedback from practitioners engaged in being critically reflective suggests that this is expressed in a variety of ways in their practice: the kinds of questions they ask, their preparedness to wait until something becomes clear or something new emerges, their willingness to ask about feelings, thoughts, values, what is 'taken for granted' as well as the influence of the broader context.

This attitude of being critically reflective also encourages an inclusive and holistic stance to practice. Critical reflection as defined here makes explicit the value of a holistic approach, in the sense of seeing oneself and others as social, emotional, mental, physical and spiritual beings influenced by and influencing their social context. This implies that practitioners will value all of who they are in contributing to practice and will similarly value the whole of those they are working with. It follows that this approach also enables practitioners to identify and articulate the spiritual, that is, what is meaningful for them, the fundamental values from which they either do operate or want to operate. Reconnecting with or unearthing these reminds practitioners what really matters to them, their preferred way of being in practice. This can restore or reinforce a sense of integrity about practice, central to practitioner satisfaction and sense of wellbeing even when resolution of specific issues or ethical dilemmas is not possible. Such an approach contributes Freshwater (2011b, p. 107) suggests to 'self-awareness, furthering development and providing a foothold towards the elusive concept of self-actualization, or perhaps more specifically, to understand and reach our personal potential in professional development'.

Second, this book offers a clearly articulated theoretical approach to being critically reflective, including how related theories can complement the key theories underlying critical reflection. The theoretical base for being critically reflective outlined here has three aspects.

First is the four key underlying key theories of critical reflection: reflective practice, reflexivity, postmodernism and critical social theory. There is considerable confusion in the literature about how to define 'reflective practice', 'reflection', 'reflexivity' and 'critical reflection' (Fook, White and Gardner, 2006). These differences and the definition of critical reflection used in this book are explored fully in Part I: Introducing Critical Reflection Theory and Processes, specifically in Chapter 1. Each of these four key theories has its own distinctive set of concepts and together these provide an integrated way of distinguishing the framework for being critically reflective advocated here. The combination of ideas using these four key theories essentially suggests that practice is always influenced by social context and complex interactions between the social context and all that each person brings to that, including their assumptions and values, which may be conscious or unconscious. Each of the theories and how they strengthen and/or complement each other is explored in Chapter 2.

Secondly, these key critical reflection theories can be complemented by other theories and some organizations use particular ones such as a strengths, narrative or psychodynamic approach. A variety of writers have also made such connections; Stedmon and Dallos (2009), for example, have chapters linking reflective practice to a range of other theories. I have chosen here to explore the use of two other relevant theories that have influenced me: psychodynamic thinking that brings a particular set of ideas for understanding the influence of what is unconscious and how this plays out in relationships. It also affirms the centrality of emotions and the influence of personal history. Partly, because of the emphasis in critical reflection on unearthing fundamental values and assumptions, I have also included current thinking about spirituality with its focus on what is meaningful, what really matters.

The third set of relevant theories relates to recognizing the influence of organizational and social contexts generally and particularly how individuals and organizations can learn and change. Professional practice generally takes place in organizations and it is crucial to understand how significantly this influences practice. Practitioners who are endeavouring to be critically reflective often see their greatest challenge as the organization they work for as opposed to the service users they work with. Managing organizational concerns is often a major issue for practice, with practitioners feeling powerless to seek change. This is particularly so in a broader social, political and economic environment of unpredictability and often diminishing resources. This relates to such issues as the pressures of rapid change and related uncertainties, the siloed nature of organizational life related to narrowly defined funding and focuses on accountability and outcomes.

Useful theories then relate to understanding organizations as systems operating within and influenced by the current political and economic context with their own cultures, sets of assumptions and values. These assumptions and values may be implicit or explicit and will play out in ways that influence practice and how organizations and practitioners interact with their particular context. Of course there is a vast array of organizational structures, philosophies, expectations and formal and informal practices. What I am suggesting here is that it is useful to see organizations both as separate entities with their own particular structure and culture, as well seeing organizations as sets of people interacting in dynamic and ever changing ways. This combination allows for both standing back to see the organization distinctly while also understanding that organizations can also be understood as people who can actively seek change. Theories about organizational learning, including transformational learning, suggest unifying these perspectives helps generate more possibilities for change (Cranton and Taylor, 2012). This, in turn, is fostered by a critically reflective attitude to understanding organizational life – unearthing the assumptions underlying the organizational culture and to what degree these match the assumptions and values of practitioners. Critical reflection can also be used as a process to reflect on or 'research' or evaluate organizational practice as a form of organizational learning. In Part II: Critical Reflection in Organizations, ideas about the current context and related issues influencing organizations are explored (Chapter 4) and related theories of organizational life and learning and possibilities for change (Chapter 5).

Finally, what is distinctive about this book is generating ideas about how to apply being critical reflective in practice. The expectation is that reflecting and practicing are inextricably linked. Schön (1983, p. 280) identifies a perception that too much reflection will be immobilizing; rather he suggests:

> in actual reflection-in-action … doing and thinking are complementary … Each feeds the other, and each sets boundaries for the other. It is the surprising result of action that triggers reflection and it is the production of a satisfactory move that brings reflection temporarily to a close.

What is necessary then is for individuals to find ways that help develop the capacity to *be* critically reflective – to reflect in action as well as after action. What I think can help here is suggesting a range of possible ways to *do* critical reflection. I want to emphasize here that these are only possibilities. I have suggested these because they are generally ones either I have used myself with individuals or groups or have known others who have used and evaluated them. However, practitioners find their own ways to be and do critical reflection adapting processes to suit their context and preferences. Some practitioners work in solo practice, some in private practice and others in a range of smaller and larger funded organizations. What is important is to find your own preferred ways of supporting a critically reflective stance.

Some organizations do actively encourage and support the use of critical reflection usually in individual or group supervision. Others don't for a variety of reasons, philosophical, financial and/or resource related and it may well be that individuals need to generate their own ways of being critically reflective. Related to this I have suggested a new way of thinking about supervision that suggests practitioners can make active choices about how to meet their needs for support and education and particularly for developing and maintaining a critically reflective attitude to practice (Chapter 6). Traditional ways of thinking about supervision are identified: the combination of accountability, support and educational roles in a one-to-one relationship between a more senior staff member and a more junior one. Instead, thinking about supervision as how professional practice is effectively supported can lead to more flexible and creative arrangements. The aim here is to encourage practitioners to think more broadly about their own assumptions about how they are supervised and how they are supported to be critically reflective in their organization and what their preferences might be. It may be that there are ways of doing this that suit both the individual and the organization. If not, this way of thinking about supervision reinforces finding your own ways to be supported in being critically reflective, which may mean creatively seeking options within or outside the organizational context.

To address this, Chapter 3 will outline many ways of using critically reflective processes, in the hope of encouraging readers to find what suits them or to feel inspired to create their own forms of doing critical reflection. I have begun with the Fook and Gardner's (2007) two-stage model for exploring specific experiences, setting out the approach in detail here, so that the key ideas are clear for those who will need to critically reflect on their own as well as those who may use critical reflection in a variety of ways with other people. The diagrams outlining the two stages suggest four possible steps with related possible questions. Stage One has three steps: (1) exploring the experience from your own perspective; (2) the perspective of the 'other' someone else in the experience or able to relate to it; and (3) articulating where you are now coming from. In Stage Two, new perspectives are identified and how these might lead to changed perspectives or actions is explored.

A number of other ways of doing critical reflection is identified that can be used individually and/or with others. These include journaling and using visual images, creating images or symbols, meeting with others in pairs or small groups, face to face or online, in blogs or email. Overall, the aim here is to affirm that there are many ways to be critically reflective, not one right way.

Understanding how to apply critical reflection is the focus of the third part of the book (Critical Reflection in the Broader Professional Context). Each of the chapters in this part takes a theme of organizational life, outlines some of the current thinking related to the theme and how practitioners might use critical reflection to engage with it. Chapter 7 outlines concerns about ethical issues and how to manage them, what some writers name as issues of morality or integrity or of moral distress and the need for moral courage. Not all such issues can be resolved. Writers agree that what can help is the use of reflective processes to engage constructively and creatively with such dilemmas, clarifying issues and related values, so that conscious choices can be made about whether and/or how to act or to manage living with such dilemmas.

Managing change, uncertainty and conflict (Chapter 8) are considered here as inevitable aspects of organizational life. The rate of change in organizations and society generally means that practitioners often feel they are living with constant uncertainty. Conflict may emerge connected to these or other issues. When uncertainty becomes real specific change, practitioners will face different challenges. Being critically reflective encourages the identification of individual and organizational assumptions about change, uncertainty and conflict that may or may not be helpful and the articulation of the influence of power, meaning and context in order to make conscious choices about whether and/or how to act.

Similar processes can also be helpful in the dynamics of interprofessional practice: the expectation of being able to work effectively with those from other professional backgrounds either within or between organizations (Chapter 9). One of the benefits of using a critically reflective approach is that it is increasingly seen as part of professional practice. Disciplines generally have a distinctive language, but with common training and agreement about how critical reflection is understood, interprofessional practitioners can use critical reflection as a shared language. The process of critical reflection can also help with identification of different professional assumptions and what these might mean for effective teamwork. Again, it helps to uncover assumptions: where might the other disciplines/agencies be coming from? What different assumptions and values are they operating under and what are the implications for practice?

Implicit in all of these is the issue of engaging with the complexity of issues of power in professional practice and particularly in relation to organizational context. Being critically reflective means understanding and engaging with how power is operating in a given experience, but also being open to new possibilities for perceiving and using power, making active choices about whether and how to act. This is not to suggest it is always possible for practitioners to resolve challenging issues individually or organizationally, but rather to see more clearly the complexity of issues of power and to make conscious and creative choices about possible strategies.

Finally, I aim to make the application of critical reflection clear by using many examples of practitioners using critical reflection throughout this book. These all originated in workshops or supervision and I have aimed to keep the style of the person relating their experience. However, to maintain confidentiality I have significantly altered details while retaining the essence of the issues and clarity that emerged. So, if you think you recognize a particular experience, it is more likely to be someone else's – and that I have so changed the original version that it now is closer to your own! There are, of course, patterns in the examples raised in workshops and I have also chosen examples that are representative of the issues raised.

In Part I, summaries of examples are used throughout the chapters. In Parts II and III, at the end of chapters, I have frequently written the examples following the Fook and Gardner (2007) two-stage critical reflection process outlined at the beginning of Chapter 3 to demonstrate the range of contexts in which it can be used. The examples at the end of each chapter illustrate the chapter's themes, so the format does vary depending on the chapter. It has been, of course, impossible to represent the vast array of examples and issues that emerged in workshops, so it is important to think about how you might apply the questions and explorations to experiences of your own. You may find that you react in a particular way to these examples – and not necessarily in the same way as the person whose experience in being presented. You can use this as an opportunity to reflect on your own practice: how might you have reacted in a similar situation? How is this similar to or different from this person? What might that mean about your underlying assumptions and values? This process will be explored in detail in chapter three.

Who might find this book useful?

In responding to questions about who might find this book useful, I have thought about how I have used the ideas and processes explored here and which groups of people have found them useful. I have used the theoretical framework and two-stage model and a range of other processes in workshops with students, newly qualified and experienced practitioners; those who are providing supervision as well as those receiving it, sometimes with a mix of all of these in a workshop. I have also had feedback, both formally and informally, on how the ideas and processes have been used. Jan Fook and I also edited a book where practitioners and researchers described a wide range of ways they had adapted the two-stage critical reflection model (Fook and Gardner, 2013). It seems that critically reflective processes and the related theoretical ideas are accessible and useful to different people in varying ways over time. Potentially then, this book may be useful for:

Students: developing the capacity to be reflective is now generally regarded as part of professional development throughout a course and particularly in clinical or field work experience. Students need tools during the initial part of their course for reflection and to begin to understand the nature of the dynamics they will have to engage with on their placements and eventually as practitioners. The material in this book can be used by students so that being critically reflective is embedded in their professional career right from the start.

Newer practitioners: the book reinforces their previous learning as students and encourages active application of critical reflection in the context of a particular organization. The approach to critical reflection and to supervision also affirms new practitioners making conscious choices about how to creatively and actively seek the kinds of support they need to be critically reflective.

Experienced practitioners (who may well also be supervisors): the theory and framework meet a range of needs depending on their level and kinds of past experience. For some, the book may reinforce and/or complement their current knowledge and skills; for others it may provide new perspectives on current theory and thinking about being critically reflective and how to relate this to practice and supervision.

Issues of language

A dilemma that arises from the interprofessional approach of this book is the use of terminology: how to name those who are engaged with services as well as those providing them. Professions and agencies have distinct preferences and often coherent arguments for their preference. Some continue to use patient or client others reject these as having implications of powerlessness. Others prefer service user or consumer to suggest a more active selector and evaluator of services or, from a person-centred approach, person or people. Some, including those working with communities, might prefer community members or simply people or always using names rather than roles or categories. I am conscious that the examples I have used are wider than users of services and how they are named depends on the particular work context. It may be individuals, families, groups or communities and may relate to direct practice, policy, research or community development. In light of this I will use the phrase service user, when appropriate, but otherwise will use person or people.

Similarly, some professional groups prefer their profession to be named, others are not so concerned. Some agencies name specific professions; others general categories of workers such as client services workers or case managers and of course these have a variety of meaning in different contexts. These terms tend to focus only on work with individuals and families and this book is also for other areas such as work with communities and in policy and program development. I have decided to use the word 'practitioner'; by which I mean someone practicing in the human services, defined broadly and inclusively. I am including students in this as 'trainee' practitioners, and am also conscious that, of course, some students are also practitioners. I name the overall fields of interest for the book as either health, education, social care or health and human services: meaning any organization that is broadly connected to working with people related to health and welfare issues. However, the processes can apply equally to other fields of practice such as law or business.

To conclude, this book encourages practitioners to develop a critically reflective attitude to their practice. Such an attitude reinforces practice that is holistic and empowering within an understanding of the influence of social context. Essentially the aim of critical reflection, as outlined here, is for practitioners to understand their own and others fundamental assumptions and values in a way that opens up possibilities for change in perspectives and actions in environments of change, uncertainty and complexity. Understanding the complexities of practice and related power dynamics can mean practitioners feel more able to generate new options and choices, making conscious decisions about whether and/or how to seek change. The two-stage process, which is outlined in detail, provides a clear and accessible framework for how to 'do' critical reflection as a way of moving towards becoming critically reflective. This and other processes outlined can be used by students as well as practitioners, individually and with others in pairs or groups or in supervision. These can also be adapted and used in a variety of creative ways to suit the particular person in their specific context.

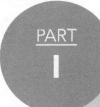

PART

I

Introducing Critical Reflection Theory and Processes

1 What is Critical Reflection?

My intention in this chapter is to outline briefly the range of current ideas or perspectives about critical reflection and reflective practice with the aim of clarifying the differences between these. In the second part of the chapter I will define how I am using critical reflection in this book, explore principles that I see as connected to being critically reflective and identify the culture of critical reflection that is the background to the examples used here.

I am conscious that interest in including reflection or critical reflection in practice has grown significantly in recent years. Professional accrediting bodies across health, human services and education now generally expect some form of reflective practice in the curriculum. Some professions, like social work (Morley, 2008; Noble and Irwin, 2009) and nursing (Johns and Freshwater, 2005; Crowe and O'Malley, 2006) have a long history of interest in being reflective; others such as allied health professions including physiotherapy, speech therapy and occupational therapy now also include reflective practice as an integral aspect of professional development (Delaney and Watkin, 2009; Cohn, Schell and Crepacu, 2010; Vachon, Durand and LeBlanc, 2010). Much current writing explores the use of reflective practice across disciplines (Fronek et al., 2009; Rolfe, Jasper and Freshwater, 2011; Oelofsen, 2012) but also in specific fields of practice such as mental health (Webber and Nathan, 2010), early childhood education (Reed and Canning, 2010), rehabilitation (Vachon, Durand and LeBlanc, 2010) working with older people (Hughes and Heycox, 2005) and in counselling (Bager-Charleson, 2010) and management (Reynolds and Vince, 2004).

Why the increased interest in reflective practice?

So why is there an increased interest in being reflective or in including reflection in practice? In the workshops Jan Fook and I have run practitioners generally experienced critical reflection as a way of developing a more complex understanding of practice that is helpful in an increasingly multifaceted and uncertain environment (Fook and Askeland, 2006). I find that

professionals in workshops often talk about the pressures of a busy and challenging workplace, where there is little time or opportunity to stop and
think, to process, to be aware of the influence of their own feelings, values
and assumptions. This combined with the challenges of working with an
increasingly diverse population reinforces their questions of how to work
with integrity as well as how to be a high-quality and effective worker. Some
would say that their impetus to be reflective is also influenced by feeling
'stuck' or challenged by situations that present moral or ethical dilemmas
(Laabs, 2011). Similarly, Lam, Wong and Leung (2007) found that 'disturbing events' were catalysts in generating critical reflection processes for social
work students.

Different approaches to critical reflection and reflective practice

What people mean by reflective practice varies considerably and this is
reflected in the sometimes bewildering range of writing about critical reflection, reflection, reflective practice and reflexivity. It is important to notice
that writers about critical reflection and reflective practice often use the
same language to talk about different things or different language to talk
about the same things (Fook, White and Gardner, 2006). This partly relates
to how the writer positions their different professional perspectives and
theoretical preferences as well as their varied experiences of being reflective
in practice and research. As a developing field, ideas about what works are
still being tested, and there is clearly a need for more research about the
effectiveness of different approaches. It is important then, when you are
reading about reflection, to seek clarity, at the outset, about what the writer
specifically means. Some writers see reflective practice and reflexivity as
essentially the same; some include critical reflection in reflective practice,
while others would see critical reflection as distinct from reflective practice.
Redmond (2004) has a helpful diagram and explanatory chapter tracing
major theorists and development of ideas about reflection over time. Fook,
White and Gardner (2006) review contemporary literature and current
approaches and Fook, (2013) reviews concepts.

A key distinction to understand clearly is the difference between reflec-
tion/reflective practice and critical reflection. Schön (1983), who is generally
seen as key in the development of reflective practice, was primarily interested in professional practice and how and why it worked. The aim of reflection, for him, was to encourage practitioners to 'surface and criticize the
tacit understandings that have grown up around the repetitive experiences
of a specialized practice' (p. 61). Such questioning of what is 'taken for
granted' means the practitioner becomes 'a researcher in the practice

context' (Schön, 1983, p. 68) moving from reflecting on actions after they have happened to reflecting in action – incorporating the ability to reflect during practice. Schön with Argyris also developed the idea of single and double loop learning in order to illustrate the difference between simply changing actions in response to feedback (single loop) and changing the underlying assumptions or theories that led to the action (double loop) (Argyris and Schön, 1996).

Many writers have used Schön's ideas to build on or to explore more specifically how practitioners can become reflective from their own perspective. Freshwater (2011b, p. 106) from a nursing perspective, for example, sees reflection as a 'cyclic thought process', which she links to clinical supervision: with reflective practice as a 'way of being that comes from the relationship between reflection and clinical supervision', which helps individuals access their ways of knowing that 'are always just below the surface'. This idea of a cyclic process has been used by a variety of other writers and has similarities to an action research cycle –reinforcing Schön's view of the practitioner researching their practice. I have also found that many people relate well to Kolb's cycle, which has been particularly influential with the four stages of learning (concrete experience, reflective observation, abstract conceptualization and active experimentation) linked to preferred styles of learning (Kolb and Kolb, 2005). In theory, reflection can start at any point in the cycle, with a focus on experience and changed reactions as a result of the reflection. Although this cycle has been criticized for not recognizing cultural influences and for not doing 'justice to the complexity of human learning' (Jarvis, 2012, p. 77), it continues to be widely used.

Learning from experience

Implicit in this view of reflection is that it relates to learning from experience. Dewey (1934) is seen as the person who initially articulated the value of learning from personal experience, which is now firmly embedded in thinking about how people learn both as students and practitioners. How experience is defined here varies including learning from activities that are part of work or life: learning from specific activities in organizations, as part of more formal study or workshops, or learning from other people's experiences. Of course these are not mutually exclusive. I find that in workshops people often learn from hearing about each other's experiences as much as processing their own; some make comments like I can't believe that we have had such a similar experience, but I never thought of seeing it in the way you have. Some writers focus directly on the influence of organizations on reflection and learning. Cressey, Boud and Docherty (2006), for example, suggest the need for 'productive' reflection where organizations create opportunities in the workplace for learning and reflection on that learning for individuals, work groups and the organization more broadly. Others point out the importance of not forgetting the physicality of experience, that experience is embodied or experienced through the senses at a particular time in a specific cultural context (Jarvis, 2012). Stedmon and Dallos (2009, p.15) put this very well suggesting that learning from experience 'involves the whole person including thoughts, feelings and senses and ... that learning in this way is a holistic process and that the process of learning is influenced by the social and emotional context in which it occurs'.

The existence of stages in reflective practice

There is also a group of writers interested in how the capacity to reflect on experience changes over time, suggesting a series of stages, which may or may not be sequential. A reasonably typical example of this that can be used to other contexts is Tan and colleagues' (2010) four stages for assessing how student teachers self-reflect on teaching: (1) pre-reflection (interpretation of classroom situations without consideration of other events or circumstances); (2) surface reflection (considerations of teaching confined to tactical issues concerning ways to achieve predefined objectives and standards); (3) pedagogical reflection (teacher considers how practices are affecting students' learning and how improvements can be incorporated); and (4) critical reflection (ongoing reflection and critical inquiry on teaching taking into consideration philosophy and ideology). However, they found that only 2 percent of students reflected critically, with 67 percent being pedagogical reflectors. This reinforces that for many practitioners it is important to learn how to become reflective and that reflection will be stimulated in varying ways over time.

This is congruent with Fowler (1981), writing about the stages of spiritual formation. He links a greater capacity to be critically reflective with increasingly complex understandings of the spiritual journey, partly but not wholly related to age and development across the life span. Trelfa (2005) supports this link and suggests stages of spiritual formation have useful parallels to stages of development as a practitioner with learning to be reflective and increasingly aware of self and social context. Carroll's (2010) six level model of reflection also links changed capacity for reflection with exploring meaning at deeper levels. His levels move from 'zero reflection' through empathic, relational, systemic, self and transcendent, with this final level being 'the reflective stance that sees 'beyond' to what makes meaning and gives meaning to life. ... For many, this can be a religious or spiritual stance that reflects a philosophy or a system of meaning that already exists (e.g. Christianity, Judaism), or one that I create (my philosophy of life)

(Carroll, 2010, p. 26). However, like Carroll, most writers emphasize that people do not necessarily work through these stages or levels sequentially. My view on this is that the idea of the stages can be helpful in identifying different ways that people reflect and that these may tend to happen for some people more at particular times of their working lives than others. However, my experience is that the development of reflective capacity is not linear or mutually exclusive. This is reinforced by Hickson (2013) who found from interviews with social work practitioners that rather than thinking about a continuum of reflection, it was more helpful to think about different kinds of reflection. She uses a helpful metaphor of ponds to explore how differently people reflect, but also how people may reflect differently at different times depending on the particular issue and context. Using this metaphor allows for seeing reflection at different levels of depth and connectedness, in different contexts and times, with different people and initiated by varying kinds of events.

Thinking holistically

There are also differences in focus, partly depending on how holistic the approach is, for example, writers are more or less accepting of the place of emotion and the interaction between the personal and the professional. Rolfe (2011a, p. 15) for example, emphasizes that critical reflection focuses on 'the transformation of the way that practitioners view the world and their place in it … what we *do* rather than who we *are*'. He is somewhat critical of what he sees as Johns' inclusion of personal learning and development; Johns (2005a) expresses concern about the increasing dominance of a rational approach to critical reflection, rather than 'reflection as a mindful, holistic and intuitive lens to view self' that offers a 'way of paying attention, of opening the doors of perception' (Johns, 2005b, p. 7). He goes on to say that '[w]e may thus become mindful of each unfolding experience in such a way as to enable us to learn from that experience and move towards realizing more desirable and satisfactory lives' (Johns, 2005b, p. 11). Johns, like others (Mezirow, 2000; Sawn and Bailey, 2004) affirm the centrality of the emotional in critical reflection: recognizing and engaging with feelings that arise from the experiences being reflected on as well as the process itself. Certainly my experience of the critically reflective process is that it is vital that people recognize and engage with their emotional reactions.

Sawn and Bailey (2004) usefully point out that emotions arise in many ways and can both generate reflection and be generated by reflection. They suggest there is a danger of critical reflection being seen as a way of managing and controlling emotions in organizations rather than as a source of organizational as well as individual change. Armstrong and Huffington

(2004, p. 3) also support the need for organizational understanding and suggest the value of a shift from seeing emotions as disturbing, 'to understanding the emotional undertow of people's experience in organizational life as a source of intelligence into the challenges and dilemmas they are facing'.

Different meanings of 'reflexivity' and 'critical'

Understanding what is meant by reflexivity also varies. For Rolfe, this connects with action: reflexivity then is questioning what is impeding or encouraging action. '[I]f the practitioner who reflects on action is *reflective*, then the one who reflects in action is a *reflexive* practitioner ... reflection-in-action can be seen as a form of practical experimentation or action research' (Rolfe, 2011b, p. 163). Stedmon and Dallos (2009, p. 4) have a related view, using '*personal reflection* to refer to the spontaneous and imme-diate act of reflecting in the moment ... to describe reflection in action ... In contrast, we use *personal reflexivity* to refer to the act of looking back over, reflecting *on* action'. This is a somewhat different emphasis to Freshwater's (2011a, pp. 185–6), who says:

> from a *critical* standpoint, reflexivity involves researchers locating them-selves within political and social positions, so that they remain mindful of the problematic nature of knowledge and power inherent in human relationships and organizations (Freshwater and Rolfe, 2001). Critical reflexivity draws particularly on the ... critical theory school of philoso-phy ... which calls into question the socio-political structures in which we all find ourselves, and which reflects particularly on the effects of power, oppression and disempowerment.

Bager-Charleson (2010) supports this view: 'Critical reflexivity involves questioning our relationship to our own culture. It concerns the link between us and our social structure.' This certainly fits better for me with the ideas of being critically reflected developed for this book.

Writers also vary in what they mean by 'critical'. Brookfield (2005, p. 11) who links 'critical' firmly to critical social theory (discussed in the next chapter), comments 'how the term critical is used inevitably reflects the worldview and ideology of the user'. For example, Crawford (2012, p. 171), says 'reflection becomes more critical and more effective where it also takes account of research and literature-based knowledge' and that more gener-ally, being critical means being 'open, honest and thoughtful' (p. 120). Bager-Charleson (2010, p. 10) acknowledges the value of 'critical friends'; 'someone, such as a trustworthy friend or colleague, who understands where you are coming from and is able to throw new light on a situation and assist you with your "blind" spots'. On the other hand Thompson and Thompson (2008, pp. 26–7) take the view that it is not appropriate to make a distinction between reflective practice and critical reflection 'as, in our view, an approach to reflective practice that does not adopt a critical perspective would produce poor quality practice and, in some respects, dangerous practice – for example, by unwittingly reinforcing patterns of discrimination'. Their view of 'critical' includes looking at both 'depth', what is happening underneath the surface, and 'breadth', the influence 'of a more holistic social and political picture at the macro level'.

More often, writers do make constructive distinctions between kinds of reflection to reinforce the point that people do reflect differently and that some people, of course will use different kinds of reflection at different times. Ghaye and Lilyman (2000, p. 13) suggests reflective practice is 'about valuing what we do and why we do it' by 'linking theory and practice and making connection with meaningful work based on authenticity, intentionality, sensibility and spirituality ... a deep sense of obligation, commitment and moral purpose' (p. 36). They contrast this with critical reflection that questions accepted routines, and also see critical as referring to practice within larger political and professional systems. Some writers would suggest that reflection is not critical enough. Reynolds and Vince (2004, p. 5) suggest that reflection in organizations is too individual and not sufficiently critical; that 'experience – the focus for reflection – has been cast in a way which takes insufficient account of its social, organizational and cultural nature'.

Reflective practice, reflexivity and critical social theory all have their own theoretical backgrounds, which are explored in more detail in the next chapter with postmodernism as the four main underlying theories for being critically reflective.

Defining being critically reflective

In this book is I am focusing on *being critically reflective*, the capacity to be reflective and to understand how that reflection is influenced by social context. Here, what distinguishes critical reflection from reflective practice or reflection is the inclusion of a *critical* approach: that what is happening in the broader society or culture will inevitably influence practice. I am conscious that for some, or perhaps many, people, the word 'critical' is unfortunate, having connotations of being judged or criticized. However, in the sense used here 'critical' affirms the link to critical social theory – seeing the influence of social context, which I will explore in detail in the next chapter. The culture of critical reflection stresses the importance of creating an atmosphere that is accepting and non-judgemental so that people feel able to explore at a deeper level how they are feeling and what they are thinking. This is essential given the process encourages being vulnerable by sharing experiences that are generally at least puzzling, but may well be uncomfortable or painful. The 'ground rules' or culture of critical reflection make explicit this expectation of not judging the other. Neither is the process about being critical in the sense of being analytical, although clearly being able to analyse in the sense of being able to explore, consider and be thoughtful is an important part of the process. If critical reflection is being supported within organizations, it is vital to ensure this enabling and accepting culture is embedded in the process, so that it isn't undermined by expectations of performance or being seen as 'surveillance, inquisition and a form of required 'confessional' (Stedmon and Dallos, 2009, p. 4).

Critical reflection here then is both a theory and a process that 'involves a deeper look at the premises on which thinking, actions and emotions are based. It is critical when connections are made between these assumptions and the social world as a basis for changed action' (Fook and Gardner, 2007, p. 14). From a holistic critical perspective, emotions, thoughts, assumptions, values and actions connected to experience are important sources of information about what is meaningful for a particular person. What is meant by assumptions here is what is 'taken for granted', our often unconscious beliefs about how things are or 'should' be. In the process of critically reflecting such assumptions become conscious and then may be affirmed and used more actively or modified or changed if not reflecting the person's preferred values and beliefs. The expectation of change is also implicit in critical reflection, specifically, change that is based on values of social justice.

Critical reflection then can be thought of as a way of understanding and engaging with interconnections between:

- an experience (and it helps the process to use a specific experience);
- the emotions, thoughts, reactions and actions related to that experience;
- meaning: what matters about the experience, including related assumptions and values at a fundamental level; and
- the influence of social context and history both individually and collectively with the expectation of the critically reflective process leading to socially just change.

Seeing critical reflection in this way makes explicit the underlying connectedness between all of these aspects of the self and of the self in relation to the social context. Generally, reflecting critically starts with an experience, which helps ground the reflection. You might also start at another point – with a sense of unease, for example, or discomfort. Alternatively, you might have a feeling of values being disconnected from your practice and ask where is this coming from? You might then connect this to a specific experience to explore more deeply where this feeling comes from and what it means in relation to values and beliefs. You could begin by considering something general like the influence of a new policy, then connect to a specific experience of the policy and your reactions to it. Possible processes for this are outlined in Chapter 3.

A holistic approach to practice is therefore also integral to being critically reflective and specifically connects to the 'being' aspect. This suggests creating an inner space that allows the dialogue of reflection: validating sitting with and paying attention to what emerges, asking about what emotions and thoughts are influencing reactions, what values and assumptions are surfacing that need to be taken into account, all within the context of the person's own history and their own and the broader social context. From a holistic perspective

> The critical reflection process requires workers to use all of themselves, to take into account the emotional, social, mental, physical and spiritual. The process is one that includes recognizing and working with emotions and thoughts, recognizing the influence of social context and the physical world and the impact of what is meaningful. (Gardner, 2011, pp. 70–1)

For Ruch (2005, p. 116) 'a recurrent feature of holistically reflective practitioners is their integration of these personal, propositional and process knowledges and their ability to constantly exercise professional curiosity and ask the question "why?" In relation to their practice'. For example, a practitioner confronted with how a 90 year old is treated in the health system might need to sit with their own inner reactions about what it means to be older, how life is valued and how this is influenced by the broader culture. If there is a question of a major operation such as a heart transplant, questions might be asked about the desirability of this at a conscious or unconscious level such as: how long will this person live? or 'is it worth doing this? Implicit in this is the cultural expectation about it being better to allocate such resources to people who will be more useful/live longer. Practitioners and clients are likely to be influenced by their own experience – perhaps of knowing an active 95 year old. The underlying assumptions compete and it helps to make them conscious, so that informed and aware choices are more likely.

Being critically reflective also assumes that there will be a readiness to work with specific experiences such as these in order to be able to understand practice more deeply. The literature on learning and professional practice acknowledges that people learn in different ways. Professional education has traditionally focused on a combination of intellectual development and practice experience. The attitude to learning implicit in using critical reflection particularly values the capacity to learn from experience. Particular assumptions underpin this kind of learning such as mistakes are useful for learning. This is not to exclude the relevance of theoretical perspectives, but to balance and integrate these with paying attention to learning from experience. As Morley (2008, p. 409) identifies students, like practitioners, need both skills but also 'an understanding that the theoretical frameworks that we draw upon, consciously or not, actually inform how we assess a person's situation, how we conceptualize what the issues may be and ultimately determine our actions in response'.

Principles for being critically reflective

So what might be useful principles for or attitudes towards being critically reflective? I have named the following principles in relatively simple ways to encourage integrating them into an attitude of being critically reflective. This is not to imply that any of these are easy to use when faced with the complexity of everyday practice. They have emerged from my experience of working with individuals and groups using critical reflection over many years, so reflect practice experience as well as being congruent with the theory of critical reflection explored in the next chapter. Implicit in all of these is first working holistically, seeking to integrate all of who you are with your practice. Second, it is also implicit that being critically reflective means approaching practice (or life) with being prepared to be patient, to pay attention to or sit with the surprising and sometimes painful emotions and aspects of practice to allow new understanding to emerge.

Actively remembering or engaging with what really matters

This sounds relatively simple, but, in practice, practitioners often describe how challenging it is in complex situations to identify what is really at the heart of what is happening. It is easy to get distracted. Sometimes this is because of the complexity of the issues and events facing particular service users or communities, and their own mixed feelings and thoughts about these. However, equally it can be the practitioner feeling overwhelmed and finding it hard to identify the fundamental values and assumptions that they want to underpin their work. For both the practitioner and the service user, the organizational expectations and constraints add to the fog of confusion. The question is how to maintain a sense of integrity in practice to be able to consciously and actively identifying the key values in a situation and how to work with them.

First then it is important to identify and engage with what really matters, that is, to do the work of understanding what is significant as a fundamental level. Second it is important to take this understanding seriously and to be active about the implications for work either directly with service users, communities or for you as a practitioner or for the organization or all of these. Often this is related to recognizing and naming the contradictions and conflicts in the work role such as your vision of yourself as an enabler and helper, while limited by organizational expectations about outcomes. What is clear is that identifying what really matters can help workers discern what they are aiming for and to retain a sense of integrity about this even when achieving the ideal may not be possible. This can mean retaining some sense of power or agency in the situation.

Paula, a palliative care nurse, had worked in a large acute hospital with palliative care beds for many years. After she completed the spirituality/pastoral care training she commented that in retrospect she felt she had become overly focused on routines and organizational expectations. What really mattered to her and to the patients and their families were human interactions and she had begun to make relationship building more of a priority and was feeling much more positive about her work role, even when this generated some tension with her manager.

Practice example

Recognizing and affirming difference

Being right or seeking to be right is very strongly ingrained for those of us in Western culture and to some degree in professional practice. We see a professional qualification as equating to a level of expertise expected by particular service users and organizations. This reinforces an underlying assumption of 'rightness' or power differences that may actually be unhelpful for a particular individual or community. We take much for granted about how we do things in all sorts of ways in our public and private life from how to connect with our clients to how decisions are made in our families. One of the aims of critical reflection is to identify our own underlying assumptions and values and in the process recognize that other people have equally valid, but different assumptions and values. In exploring a particular experience, participants in critical reflection processes may see the need to move from an assumption of 'my way is the right way' to: 'my way is not the only right way'; 'there are many ways'; or 'different ways will suit different people'.

To truly affirm difference, as practitioners, we need to develop the capacity to stand back from our own preferences about how things should be done to allow and affirm the value of how other people approach doing the same things. This can be as simple as different assumptions about what to wear to work or as complex as assumptions related to death and dying. The attitude of being critically reflective can generate a sense of frequent surprise at what we take for granted. It is important in being critically reflective to move from tolerating difference to actively celebrating being different, that is, acknowledging that we are all different from each other, not that everyone else is different from me.

> **Practice example**
>
> Tanya, for example, had left a job that she had been passionately committed to. In the end, she also felt exhausted by it and decided to move to another job in the same organization with fewer hours. A new worker, Sarah, was appointed and Tanya had a week's handover with her. After that initial week, Tanya continued to drop in to see how Sarah was going and to make suggestions about what her priorities should be. Eventually, Sarah became frustrated and told Tanya that she wanted her to leave her do to the job the way she wanted to and that she didn't want to 'burn out' as Tanya had. Tanya felt quite hurt by Sarah's reaction. When she critically reflected on this, she realized that her assumption was that 'my way is the best way to do this job'. She acknowledged that her approach had worn her out and that she couldn't sustain it in practice. This led to a several new assumptions: 'there are many ways to do this job effectively'; 'my way was not sustainable'; 'I need to acknowledge the value of my passion and commitment, but work in ways that I can manage'.

A sense of openness and creativity

Another aspect of being critically reflective is having an attitude of openness. As practitioners, we generally expect this of ourselves in a general sense, but find it difficult to maintain when feeling beleaguered by demanding workloads. The desire to be open is often undermined by the pressure for closure, efficiency or the awareness of a waiting list or other work expectations. This lessens the capacity to be creative and to look for new ways that might work better for particular people. This sense of openness also means listening for what really matters to an individual, not making assumptions based on initial contact or other people's views. It requires coming to each person or situation with a freshness and readiness to engage with them, rather than being overly influenced by past experience. This is not to negate the value of professional experience in the development of knowledge, but to recognize the danger of reacting from that experience rather than from the person that you are currently engaged with. Ideally, it is as if you are responding as if this was the first time, with your knowledge and experience in the background rather than the foreground.

Sally, is a relationship counsellor who had been working with couple and families for many years. She realized that she had begun to categorize couples when they arrived in relation to the possibilities for remaining together. One day she was surprised that a particular couple she had been sure would separate, said they were feeling so much more positive they had decided to go on a long holiday together. In reflecting on her surprise, she wondered whether the couple had managed this in spite of her rather than because her. She recognized that her feelings of over familiarity with this work might well be getting in the way and that something needed to change.

Practice example

Holding opposites in creative tension

Western culture encourages thinking in binaries or dichotomies, pairs of opposites in which one is perceived as better than the other, more powerful, more able, in some way superior. Eastern culture tends to be more able to simply live with contradictions. Dichotomous thinking limits our ability to be creative: we are too busy trying to decide which of the pairs of opposites is the appropriate one rather than seeing there are many choices. Being critically reflective suggests an attitude of mind that is about allowing for possibilities that are not necessarily consistent. Most of us, for example, would have contradictory assumptions and sometimes values. What can help is simply to 'be' or 'sit' with these until we reach clarity about our preference or become comfortable about living with the contradictions, for example, wanting to live at the beach, but also in in an inland city. Sometimes identifying a range of contradictory possibilities allows or frees up thinking about how things could be or creates a completely new idea.

Patrick, an occupational therapist, worked in a small rural community health setting. His experience was of feeling immobilized by his contradictory feelings about a particular family with a child with a significant disability. On the one hand, he believed that parents should make their own choices about how they used his time, on the other hand, he felt he should be making more progress with the child's specific issues, rather than primarily talking with the parent about her experience of having a child with a disability. Is it, he asked, more important to do what she wants or am I right in thinking I should be doing something else? Will the parent be more able to manage the child well if I listen to her more? As he talked more about the family and the dilemma he saw that he was getting too focused on seeing only these options and that he was also assuming it was his decision alone. He decided to suggest to the parent that they brainstorm as a family what they would like to be using his time for and this generated new possibilities that meant the parent and the child's needs were met.

Practice example

Seeking connectedness as well as valuing difference

Being critically reflective is also about seeking connections as well as valuing difference. In Western culture, we tend to emphasize distinctiveness, uniqueness, individuality often with implications of greater power and influence. Eastern cultures tend to be more comfortable with overlap, synchronicity, what is shared or common between individuals and cultures. In the West, practitioners stress discrete aspects of life, boundaries and neatness of divisions and categories. While of course there are distinct aspects of life, it is also enabling to see when it is more accurate to talk about the complex links and interactions that create commonalities. While it may or may not be helpful as a professional to share aspects of your personal life with another person, it is often significant to recognize and validate the commonness of the human experience. Being able to empathize with another person is partly about being able to recognize the similarities as well as the differences, a more egalitarian connection.

> **Practice example**
>
> Tammy started work in palliative care feeling very conscious of her own recent, sudden and painful loss of her father. Because of that she wanted to make clear that she was operating as a competent and professional in control of her life generally and particularly her emotions. Her incident was about feeling hurt by a service user's comment about her cold and remote manner. As she explored where they were each coming from, she realized that she was putting so much energy into looking not 'like a client' that she probably did seem remote. Having shared her fear of behaving 'unprofessionally', she suddenly understood that her assumptions about being professional no longer fitted with what she saw as important in a professional role. Showing emotion, for example, might be equally helpful to clients. She decided that it would be better for her and her clients for her to acknowledge at least to herself, and if appropriate to them, their shared vulnerability and that being empathic did not exclude being competent.

Willingness to learn from experience

This particular attitude means being prepared to actively seek the meaning of a particular experience. Part of the expectation here is that critically reflective practitioners will be open to challenging themselves in a positive way, seeking opportunities to delve more deeply into the meaning of a particular experience in order to understand it a more fundamental level. Some people who have been working with critical reflection for some time say there are particular themes that emerged from their critical reflections. As they have engaged with this over time, their understanding of how this particular way of reacting has developed often deepens. This can then lead to a clearer sense of how to act differently – it may be, for example, that the person understands more fully what the issue is and so what action will be effective.

Greg's experience involved a colleague, Ben, criticizing him for being arrogant, because he had told Ben how differently he should approach his work. Greg completely disagreed with this, saying he thought it was reasonable to put another point of view about how things should be done – particularly since he was more experienced. The group asked Greg what he understood as the definition of being arrogant, which he found hard to do, so he asked the group to generate ideas about what they associated with being arrogant. One of the group members said 'pushy', 'keeping on telling you things when you've got the message, but don't agree'. This was an 'ouch' moment for Greg: he volunteered that he had had similar comments in the past, including from his partner. He decided he needed to think more about how he made suggestions.

Practice example

Linking to context and history and the influence of power

The critical aspect of critical reflection relates to taking into account a person's own social and cultural history as well as understanding how they have been influenced by the broader social context and history. People internalize the assumptions from their individual and collective situations, which affects their perceptions of their own capacity for power and influence. Being gay, for example, is likely to be experienced differently in 2011 compared to 1970 depending on where you live: the general culture has changed and this in turn has changed attitudes in families, which have in turn influenced attitudes in the general culture. Being critically reflective means engaging with the complexities of what this might mean, being prepared to ask what the person's own personal experiences related to history might be and also how these might be mediated by the cultural environment in which they live. For professionals in professional practice, organizations are also influenced by the prevailing culture and continue to influence it in their turn. The organizational culture then also needs to be taken into account in thinking about context and history.

Culture of critical reflection

As will be clear from the examples used above, critical reflection can be challenging at many levels, personally and professionally, as well as stimulating, revelatory and inspiring. My experience of using critical reflection is that it works best when there are clear expectations and the establishment of appropriate culture, whether you are using the processes on your own, with another individual or in a group, in supervision or informally.

Critical reflection is first and essentially a non-judgemental process: the aim is not to be making comments about whether someone did, thought or felt something that was 'right' or 'wrong', or appropriate or not. The expectation is that the person has brought a particular experience to the reflection because they want to understand more deeply something about it. Usually, this experience is something that is already puzzling, bothering or concerning them. Being critical in the sense of making judgements is therefore not helpful, but it is also not helpful to be simply reassuring them. If the incident is clearly upsetting, it is, of course appropriate to be empathic, but also to bear in mind that the person bringing the incident has decided they want to explore it.

From this perspective, the culture of critical reflection focuses on exploration, what a narrative approach might name as maintaining a 'stance of curiosity' (Morgan, 2000). The expectation is to keep asking why, assuming that there are likely to many reasons why, not just one. I find that not everyone likes the word why, some feel it implies a judgement. This is why in the sense of: where were you coming from when …?; what influenced you to …?; how did you come to …?; What were you feeling when …? The aim is to help the person find clarity for themselves about the *meaning* of the experience for *them* – which may well be quite different from what someone else might expect.

Acceptance is the somewhat paradoxical next key aspect of a culture of critical reflection: that the person was doing what seemed reasonable at the time or being what felt like the only way they could be. At the same time, given critical reflection's postmodern underpinnings, there is the expectation that there are always other ways, other possibilities and part of the process is about unearthing these. Sometimes this feels quite confronting, so it is important that it is done in a spirit of what are the other possibilities, not what would have been better to do.

Given the nature of the experiences people may want to explore, it is of course vital that discussions remain confidential. Sometimes the person sharing the experience may also reinforce this by altering details. However, there are times, especially in teams using critical reflection over time, when others will also know about a particular experience and who else was involved in it. If this is the case, it is important, both to affirm confidentiality in general, but to also remember that only one side of the story is being presented and not to allow the discussion to affect other relationships outside the group.

Finally, in critical reflection, because the discussion of an experience can raise unexpected emotions and new understandings it is important that the person presenting the experience be the one who has ultimate control of the process: to ask, for example, for the rate of questions to slow down or to say that they want to stop and take time to think about, on their own, what has emerged.

Summary

Critical reflection, reflective practice, reflection and reflexivity are defined quite differently in the literature. This book is focusing on critical reflection: defined as a way of understanding and engaging with interconnections between:

- an experience;
- the emotions, thoughts and reactions and actions related to that experience;
- meaning: what matters about the experience, including related assumptions and values at a fundamental level; and
- the influence of social context and history both individually and collectively with the expectation of the critically reflective process leading to socially just change.

This definition is underpinned by four main theoretical approaches: reflective practice and reflexivity as well as critical theory and postmodernism, which will be explored in the next chapter.

- What language would you have used to talk about reflecting on practice?
- What is your reaction to the definition of critical reflection used here?
- What do you think has influenced your reaction?
- What beginning thoughts and feelings do you have about the suggested culture of critical reflection?

Questions for reflection

2   Theoretical Underpinnings

There are many theoretical frameworks that can contribute to being criti-cally reflective. The main aim of this chapter is to detail the four theories that Jan Fook and I have used as the primary underpinning blocks for crit-ical reflection (Fook and Gardner, 2007). Practitioners and their organiza-tions also often have particular theories they use to complement critical reflection, such as a psychodynamic or narrative approach (Stedmon and Dallos, 2009). To illustrate how this might be done, I will also explore how understandings of psychodynamic theory and of spirituality and meaning relate to these theories: where they complement and reinforce them and/or where they differ. Why this particular combination? This reflects my own interests and preferences. Both personally and professionally, I use the theories from critical reflection complemented by psychodynamic and spirituality theory, and find them an effective combination of ideas for thinking about my own practice, in running critical reflection workshops, supervision and critical reflection workshops, and supervision and spiri-tuality workshops of various kinds. In this chapter, I will briefly summa-rize these approaches, then focus on the four main theories of critical reflection, including psychodynamic and spirituality theory and their contribution.

Summary of the four key theories

These will be described in more detail in this chapter, but an initial overview follows:

- *Reflective practice*: emphasizes identifying the feelings, thoughts, values and assumptions that influence practice; valuing experiential or practice knowledge and developing awareness of the differences between espoused theory and theory used in practice.
- *Reflexivity*: generates understanding about the complexities of how workers and their service users/communities perceive themselves and each other, the value of understanding that all of who we are

(physically, emotionally, mentally, socially, spiritually) influences how we perceive others and are perceived by them.

- *Postmodernism*: challenges modernist thinking that assigns people to limiting categories and often to binaries, understanding of the impact of current thinking at a social level including attitudes to and influences of power and how this is embedded in language.
- *Critical social theory*: identifies the interrelationships between cultural and social values and expectations and how these are internalized by individuals, often in unhelpful ways; emphasizes importance of social justice approach.

Linking to a psychodynamic approach

The four theories summarized above reinforce the importance of bringing what we are not aware of into awareness, making what is unconscious, conscious. In reflective practice, the expectation is that practitioners will articulate 'taken for granted' influences on their practice. The 'critical' in critical reflection refers to critical social theory, which clarifies the value of making conscious values and attitudes that have been internalized and so become an unconscious and potentially damaging part of practice: 'it describes the process by which people learn to recognize how uncritically accepted and unjust dominant ideologies are embedded in everyday situations and practices' (Brookfield, 2000, p. 128).

A psychodynamic approach can foster understanding of the range of ways we guard against recognizing what is painful or what we do not want to be aware of. This approach has what I think is helpful language, to make explicit various ways to think about unconscious material, naming different aspects of being unaware. For example, Johnson (1993) explores Jung's (1968) concept of the 'shadow' as the parts of ourselves that are less acceptable to us, the aspects that we push into the unconscious. These may be qualities that we value but do not see ourselves as having or alternatively parts of ourselves that we do not value but fear that we have. For example, I might wish I could emulate another person's clarity without recognizing or accepting my own. Understanding these different possibilities of what is unconscious can help with exploring reactions to a particular experience. Writers like Huffington and colleagues (2004) and Vince (2002) also suggest that this is useful from an organizational perspective: that organizations are adept at ignoring what is happening at an unconscious level particularly emotionally and that this can significantly affect organizational dynamics. Examples of these are given, later in the chapter.

Writers vary in their views about how critical reflection and psychodynamic thinking relate. Mezirow (2000, p. 23), for example, says:

Critical reflection in the context of psychotherapy focuses on assumptions regarding feelings pertaining to interpersonal relationships, in adult education its focus is on an infinitely wider range of concepts and their accompanying cognitive, affective and somative dimensions. This distinction is important in differentiating between these two professional fields.

This focus on interpersonal relationships Brookfield (2005) suggests enables the identification of childhood traumas based on assumptions that can then be reappraised. Whether or not there is trauma, both affirm that personal history, including family patterns continues to influence individuals. These need to be made conscious and often changed. Part of what is common in both approaches (critical social theory and psychodynamic thinking) is recognizing that 'such subjective reframing commonly involves an intensive and difficult emotional struggle as old perspectives become challenged and transformed' with new understandings leading to 'taking action on reflective insights' (Mezirow, 2000, pp. 23–4). Here psychodynamic thinking usefully names the 'defences' used to avoid or resist this struggle such as denial or resistance.

Ruch (2009) articulates the value of a relationship-based reflection model originating from a psychodynamic approach, which she sees as having commonalities and potential compatibilities with critical reflection. She, like Mezirow (2000) and Brookfield (2005), agrees that critical reflection more clearly articulates the 'critical' or structural and also the need for action and change. She suggests that a relationships-based model prioritizes more clearly the need for a safe space for this depth of reflection given the emotions likely to be expressed, (although she acknowledges the culture of critical reflection outlined in the Fook and Gardner (2007) model) and is more accepting of a therapeutic dimension to reflection. However, there is also some recognition in psychodynamic writing of a critical perspective. Moodley, Gielen and Wu (2013, p. 5) suggest that those using psychodynamic thinking in counselling and psychotherapy have been empowered by the 'civil rights struggles and subsequent movements seeking liberation from economic and political discrimination … to address the prevailing inequalities concerning race, culture and ethnicity in their clinical practices'.

The connection to spirituality and meaning

The literature related to spirituality and meaning can also contribute in a variety of ways to being critically reflective. First in valuing the experiential Tacey (2011, p. 194) suggests spirituality is no longer necessarily about the religious life, but rather 'the living heart of the individual and the locality of spirituality has shifted from tradition to experience'. He suggests that this 'new spirituality' can be 'accommodated by the traditional faiths, but only if they are prepared to place experience before dogma' (p. 195). Similarly, Heelas and Woodhead (2005) found that many people were interested in a more subjective sense of spirituality again with a focus on individual and inner experience. For many people then, spirituality is about their individual sense of what is meaningful to them and it helps if we can understand that as practitioners.

Second, what I mean by spirituality is that which gives life meaning including a sense of something greater or transcendent. Spirituality, in this sense, can include, but is not limited to religious beliefs. What is helpful about including spirituality in professional practice is that, like critical reflection, it focuses attention on fundamental values, on what really matters for individuals and communities, for workers as well as those they work with (Canda and Furman, 2010). This paying attention to fundamental values reinforces being critically reflective: focusing on the underlying values and assumptions that are influencing practice. This is often the place of integrity and meaning that supports practice that is confronting for practitioners.

Third, including spirituality reinforces the holistic approach implicit in being critically reflective. It is clear that many service users and communities see spirituality as an integral part of their lives whether they are refugees (Martin, 2009; Ni Raghallaigh, 2011) seeking deeper meaning related to a crisis, or simply are looking for more than a materialist attitude to life, which can include ecological concerns (Nangle, 2008). They then want that to be translated into how they engage with practitioners and agencies. White (2006, p. 40) suggests that:

> a better understanding of spirituality is the key to attempting to re-estab-lish a health service that is both holistic and effective … Both patients and staff want to work in a more holistic way; discussions about the nature of spirituality and spiritual care could help make this a reality.

The four theories underpinning critical reflection

Reflective practice

The first key theory is reflective practice, which is generally seen as originating with Schön (1983), who applied his thinking across a range of professional disciplines. He encouraged professionals to recognize the value of their own 'theories' or 'practice wisdom' in the sense of learning from their own experience as well as from more formal theoretical perspectives. This learning from experience includes the ability to stand back from what is happening to explore thoughts, reactions and/or assumptions that might be influencing a situation. Implicit in this is validating knowledge that is generated from experience and Schön (1983, p. 300) reminds practitioners working with service users that 'I am not the only one in the situation to have relevant and important knowledge' and 'My uncertainties may be a source of learning for me and for them'. This affirms that rather than the power differences of expert/service user, reflective practitioners seek connections and mutual respect. Workshop participants often reflect this. It also reminds them to validate their experience and how it has become part of their 'practice wisdom' or knowledge about how to work effectively in a given context. This can be particularly affirming in contexts where workers feel undervalued.

Focusing on the feelings or emotions is often a gateway to accessing the underlying assumptions or values that are important and that each person is reacting from. This too is central to psychodynamic thinking (Wright, 2009). It might be, for example that in an interview a practitioner becomes conscious of a feeling of irritation with the service user. From a reflective practice perspective, the practitioner would pay attention to this feeling and explore related thoughts and assumptions asking why they are feeling irritated – is what the service user is expressing contradictory to the practitioner's own values or preferred ways of being or from a psychodynamic perspective does this reflect irritation with someone else, a frustrating family member or past colleague? This can of course equally happen with colleagues or other staff in an organization. Schön's hope was that practitioners would so develop this ability that they would move from reflecting on action after the event to being able to reflect in action during the event. The ability to be reflective would become part of how the person operated. He described this as validating an intuitive and creative approach to practice, responding flexibly as needed.

Practice example

Simon was irritated by a colleague wearing a hat. While there were some logical safety reasons for this, he felt that his irritation was out of proportion. In a critically reflective process, he was able to acknowledge the influence of experiences that he had (in psychodynamic terms) repressed. He connected related painful feelings to his own history and social context: specifically coming from a different culture to the prevailing one in a small country town. His unconscious related assumption was that 'life is better for everyone if you conform to the prevailing norms' and so 'people should conform in the workplace'. The buttons being pressed by the person wearing a hat were 'why can this person get away with not conforming when I had to?' When he articulated this, he let go of the depth of irritation and was able to communicate constructively about safety issues.

Schön (1983) also articulated the difference between what he called 'espoused' theory and 'theory in practice', that is, between what a practitioner believed they were doing and what they were actually doing. Being reflective enables practitioners to check internally whether they are reacting in ways that mirror their preferred beliefs and values. This connects to thinking about the spiritual in the sense of what is meaningful, what really matters for a particular person, whether service user or a practitioner. For practitioners, this also links to what is named as working from a place of integrity or working with morality. What is common here is about wanting to work in a way that is congruent with underlying values. Given this, it is vital for practitioners to be able to name these values, to see how they might be similar to or different from those they are working with.

Practice example

Julia worked as a counsellor in a family and children's services organization, where the expectation was that the whole family would be involved in counselling. Her espoused theory was to work from a feminist perspective by which she meant that men and women were equally capable of being good parents. The experience she brought to critical reflection was about a father who felt that she was excluding him from practice with his family. As we explored this, she acknowledged that she made appointment times that were difficult for him to attend. When he did, she still addressed questions to the mother, if he responded she checked with the mother that his answer was accurate, but not with him when the mother responded. When she thought about her underlying beliefs she realized that coming from a single-parent family (with her mother) and being a single mother herself her underlying assumption was that it's always the women in the family who know what is happening. She acknowledged that at a conscious level she knew men who were active and energetic parents and what needed to change was her underlying assumptions and related actions. She worked with the group to identify how to ground her assumption that men and women are equally capable of being good parents at an emotional rather than a purely intellectual level and what this would mean about how differently she might operate in practice.

In encouraging reflection about practice, Schön also made explicit the value of a creative and intuitive approach. He suggests that knowing a particular technique or having a set of rules will not be sufficient in professional practice. What is needed is the ability to understand and translate a particular way of working in a way that will make sense to a service user given their situation. An analogy of this is knowing how to ride a bicycle in theory, but needing to learn how to ride it in practice and then how to adapt riding the bicycle to a particular surrounding. It might be for example, that as a professional you have been to a recent workshop, perhaps in narrative therapy and you now want to use this in your practice. You know the theory, you understand a specific technique and perhaps you have also practised it in workshops. Now, faced with a service user, you need to creatively adapt your understanding to suit this particular person. Schön points out that this requires a certain amount of creativity or artistry, an expectation that one way is not going to work with everyone. It further affirms a valuing of experiential knowledge, recognition that we need to pay attention to experiences and learn from them how to adapt in an intuitive way. This is also reinforced by writings about spiritual experience, that not all experiences can be rationally explained. Some might instead require an intuitive understanding or simply acceptance. A service user who says, for example, that they feel heartened by walking on the beach may simply want this validated rather than justified or explained.

Reflexivity

Reflexivity is the second key theoretical perspective. Walsh (2012, p. 192) suggests practitioners need ongoing reflection, 'a self-consciousness that allows us to be reflexive, to consider how we impact others, how we present to others, how we are perceived and that includes the context within which we engage, as well as our role and specific mandate'. The image of looking in a mirror is often helpful in understanding reflexivity. When we look in a mirror we only see relatively limited views of ourselves. In photographs, we are often surprised by how different we look – sometimes pleasantly and sometimes not. This can be a reminder that we may be perceived differently by others from the way we perceive ourselves – they are seeing different views, ones that we are not so conscious of. It then follows that we may be seeing others differently from the way they see themselves. Examples of this of course happen all the time. At one stage, in a small seminar group, I had two students who were equally apprehensive about working with each other: one was 20 and feared the relative experience and wisdom of the 50 year old; the 50 year old feared the relative energy and clarity of the 20 year old. It was only when they had to work in a pair that they recognized the assumptions each was making about the other and moved beyond them.

The idea of reflexivity asserts that all of who we are will influence how we are with others. We cannot completely separate the personal from the professional or the physical from the emotional and cultural. Who we are is embodied. We, and our service users, make assumptions about what we are like at least partly on the basis of our physical beings. This is perhaps more obvious in assumptions about gender, race and ethnicity, but equally happens in relation to how we choose to present ourselves in how we dress, the messages conveyed by hair and general appearance. When I carried out evaluation interviews for a strengths-focused organization, one of the service users commented how much difference it made having a practitioner who wore shorts and sandals rather than being formally dressed in a suit. Stedmon and Dallos (2009, p. 42) suggest a biopsychosocial approach to reflection given increased evidence from neurological studies of brain functioning of how sites in the brain develop related to the 'capacity for social cognition and, ultimately reflective functioning'.

Psychodynamic thinking related to projection and transference are useful related ways of thinking about the complexities of reflexivity. Projection is essentially when we find it easier to see a particular quality in another person rather than in ourselves. This can also happen with organizations. Andersen (2012) writes about organizations as 'projection screens'. We often think of this in a negative way, for example, seeing someone else's anger or resentment or jealousy, but this can equally apply to positive aspects of the self. Jo, for example, became conscious of how often she commented on how competent and caring her supervisor was, but that when other people congratulated her on her own competence she assumed they were being 'nice'. Transference, similarly is when, at an unconscious level, we experience a relationship in a way that relates to past relationship and make assumptions as a result. For example, a young woman working with an older woman might expect her to behave in a motherly way, positively or negatively. In counter transference the practitioner might respond to this unconscious expectation by behaving as if the other practitioner or service user is a daughter. Both then might enact their own expectations of what such a relationship might mean. Making this conscious can significantly change both this relationship and potentially others.

Reflexivity also reminds us that our personal and collective social history and context continue to influence us and we need to use these consciously rather than being swayed unconsciously (Gardner, 2012). Keenan (2012, pp. 259–60) identifies the importance of asking reflexive questions that make these connections explicit, such as: 'What socially available forms of problem definition am I invited to find compelling, promising, or productive? What socially available forms of judgement am I being invited to impose?' Understanding this is a powerful tool for professionals. It enables people to recognize how their own and others preferred ways of being have been influenced by the social context and how these might influence their practice (Freshwater, 2002). At the same time reflexivity is helpful in recognizing that what is seen as meaningful to one person is likely to be different from what is seen as meaningful to another. Parton (2007) suggests that reflexivity is at the core of social constructionism: the understanding that we all create our own social worlds and cannot then assume others will experience the world in the same way. As Iversen, Gergen, and Fairbanks (2005, p. 696) suggest 'we live in conflicting communities of the real and the good, and if we are to go on together, reflexive dialogue is essential'.

This is useful in a number of ways in practice. Perhaps the most obvious is reminding professionals to be conscious that they need to step into the shoes of the other person as much as possible in order to see how they are perceived. It is then possible, as a child protection practitioner, or a psychiatric nurse, to see that the service user is likely to be seeing what your professional label means for them rather than seeing who you are as an individual. Being able to disconnect these is very helpful in not taking personally the negative reaction of people that you might be working with. An example of mine here is working with an indigenous community when I worked for the government department responsible for removing children at risk. Although the community had requested a practitioner from the Department on a liaison committee, I was surprised to find people reluctant to engage with me. It took me quite some time to realize that I symbolized white dominant culture that had been, and continued to be, responsible for undermining the community. It was only once I recognized and accepted that, as a privileged member of the white community and a social practitioner in this government department I did share a sense of shame and responsibility, we were able to build relationships and move on (Gardner, 2012).

Postmodernism

Postmodernism is often contrasted to modernism or modernity, which is a way of looking at the world characterized by certainty; the expectation that a more scientific or positivist approach to problems will identify the cause and find the 'right' solution. This modernist approach fits with the organizational pressures to work in an outcome-focused, goal-oriented, one-size-fits-all way that can discourage being intuitive or including the beliefs and values influencing a service user's life. Postmodernism in comparison emphasizes the diversity and complexity of what influences events and a more subjective way of experiencing the world. Heelas and Woodhead's (2005) research found that many people in an English town named spirituality, as opposed to religion, as 'subjective-life' understood as 'living life with your own inner sense of authority or guidance about how to live as opposed to being guided by an external authority such as a religious body'. Postmodernism is sometimes criticized for being value free, for emphasizing subjectivity to such a degree that there can be no shared values as a basis for action. There are of course various ways of defining postmodernism. Rosenau (1992, p. 15) makes a helpful distinction between sceptical post-modernism as a period of value free 'fragmentation, disintegration, malaise, meaninglessness, a valuelessness or even absence of moral parameters and societal chaos' and what is more appropriate for practice: affirmative post-modernists 'a more hopeful, optimistic view ... (they) do not shy ... from affirming an ethic, making normative choices and striving to build issue-specific political coalitions'.

Postmodern thinking is strongly influential in Western culture and has much to offer critically reflective practice. The perspective from reflexivity that we might be seen in a variety of ways is reinforced by postmodern thinking, which suggests that all of us have 'multiple selves'; we all play many roles, and are complex human beings. From this perspective we need to think holistically about those we work with: who are they in the most general sense, what is important to them. Service users generally present at times in life when things are not going well and it can be hard to remember that there are likely to be other, resourceful and able aspects of this person.

> **Practice example**
>
> I worked as a counsellor with a man who had significant issues with alcohol use that were jeopardizing his marriage, but he also maintained a job in a senior position in a very large organization. When he came to see me he would take off his tie, turn off his mobile phone and often become visibly distressed as he talked about the impact of his alcohol use. What he wanted to talk about was not only his alcohol use and desire to do

> something about it, but also how he could believe he was worthwhile as a human being. At the end of the session he would regain his composure, put on his tie, turn on his phone and set off again looking like a competent executive.

Postmodernism also raises awareness of dichotomous thinking, that is, seeing the world in pairs of opposites, which imply that one group is better than the other (Fook, 2002). Some examples of this are parent–child; teacher–student; practitioner–service user; male–female; able–not able; and powerful–powerless. We also tend to create such acceptable and unacceptable dichotomies on a community or world scale: one cultural group is better than another; one country is right, another wrong. Having such pairs of opposites implies that there are only two ways to be rather than a multiplicity. It also tends to reinforce or create a sense of other, that is, you are either a practitioner or a service user and since it is clearly more desirable to be a practitioner, the service user is then seen as the other, the person in the less desirable position. We create this in all sorts of ways, some very subtle, often to preserve ourselves from the potential pain of being in the 'other' category.

Practice example

Patricia, who was new to child protection, was struggling to build relationships with her service users. When she explored this she realized that because of her previous financial position she had felt her own family was vulnerable to becoming a service user. Unconsciously, to reinforce her role as a practitioner she was asserting her difference from being a service user: her underlying assumption was 'I am completely different from you'. This made it very difficult to empathize with her service users and it was only when she could change her assumption to 'we have much in common' that she could engage more effectively.

Postmodernism then encourages a more holistic way of approaching practice: asking what are the multiplicity of experiences, roles, beliefs and perspectives that make up this particular person. This multiplicity generates greater uncertainty but also more possibilities. As Lartey (2003, p. 39) puts it 'The postmodern condition into which we have been ushered is characterized on the one hand by ephemerality and uncertainty – a situation that has been sharply criticized by many – and on the other hand by endless possibilities for new ways of being'. While the concept of working holistically is often appealing for professionals, there are often challenges in managing the balance between the valuing of creating possibilities and organizational expectations of specific outcomes.

Like reflexivity, postmodernism also identifies the influence of 'dominant discourses'; the main ways of thinking in contemporary culture, such as about gender, age, ethnicity, sexuality, what are the assumptions that are part of community life. Often these are contradictory and complex: for example, that everyone is equally able to achieve anything combined with the recognition that those who are wealthier have greater choices. Postmodernists also identify the dominant ways of thinking about power, but suggest that this is more complicated than it appears, that power can be exercised rather than only imposed, can be bottom up as well as top down and be repressive and productive (Healy, 2000). Often in organizations, people assume that those who are more senior will have more power and of course this is often the case. However, power is not only linked to position in the organizational hierarchy, practitioners can also be powerful on the basis of their convictions and passions, their determination, the length of time they have been in the organization and so their perceived degree of knowledge and of course by their capacity to link together for shared action. Supervisors in workshops often comment that while they are, in theory, more powerful it is very difficult to 'make' a practitioner carry out a particular activity, which they are reluctant to do.

> **Practice example**
>
> Maree worked in a finance/budgeting role in a large health organization. She was frustrated that at the end of each financial year, departments would be asked to put in budgets and the process was always rushed and led to frustration and resentment. Her specific experience related to having an argument with her line manager partly related to the stress of this. After considerable discussion, she acknowledged her assumption 'I am stuck with this'; 'I am powerless to change this', which she connected to the position of women in the organization and society. When challenged, she agreed that it was an assumption and explored the implications of a new assumption: 'I have the knowledge and skills to change this'. A plan emerged: to talk to her line manager

with a one page proposal outlining what she thought would work. She remained dubious, but to her surprise her line manager agreed to support her proposal. Her assumption shifted to seeing herself as able to raise difficult issues constructively from a position of power, given her experience and history within the organization.

Connected to all these ideas is the affirmation of diversity, a position that suggests that each individual's subjective sense of what is 'right' for them is a reasonable direction to take. This fits with the current experience of spirituality where many individuals are more likely to identify their own sense of meaning and create a network to support this, while others will continue to value the support of a religious tradition. Postmodernism also reinforces that there is always complexity of cause and therefore many possible solutions. Postmodernists generally go further than tolerance of diversity to active inclusion, particularly questioning who is being marginalized and how they can be actively included. However, it is important to recognize that postmodernists like any other group vary: some would be reluctant to suggest any kind of shared sense of culture, preferring always to ask what the subjective meaning is for a particular person.

Critical social theory

The flexibility and diversity of postmodernism can be balanced in being critically reflective with critical social theory. The 'critical' aspect of this theory is that individuals are continually interacting with, being affected by and influencing the social structures in which they live. A key aspect of critical social theory is that individuals internalize, or take on board at an unconscious level, the prevailing ideas of the culture they live in, so that there can be a form of internal oppression as well as external. Kumsa (2012, p. 319) calls this 'critical reflexivity' and takes further the view that we can unwittingly replicate the cultural oppression that we want to change. She suggests the Self may be identified as inner (and oppressed) and the 'Other' as outer (and the oppressor), but that these are actually intertwined: we need to recognize how we internalize the oppressor within, rather than always looking for external oppressors. Part of the challenge of this is how difficult it is to truly understand how it feels to be perceived as culturally different, particularly for those who are in the dominating culture. I remember hearing a story of a surgeon whose attitude to what it was like to be a patient shifted dramatically after an experience of being in hospital himself.

Fred, a black worker in car manufacturing, unemployed because of the downturn in the economy might, for example, blame himself for not seeking other educational opportunities, rather than recognizing the broader forces that have led to the redundancy. The underlying assumption might be: unemployed people have only themselves to blame and/or people are only of worth when employed; assumptions influenced by the prevailing culture about men who are black and unemployed and internalized in a way that may lead to depression, rather than recognition that some factors are beyond his control.

Practice example

The considerable writings about liberation theology also use critical social theory to explore the connections between the individual and the society in which they live. These writings are often helpfully explicit about the complexities of difference and challenges of working for a more socially just society. Sneed (2010), for example, writes about his experience of being black, gay and Christian and his struggle to have recognized that for him the combination of these is what is important rather than seeing one as primary. He advocates an 'ethic of openness' that 'goes beyond mere tolerance and involves a deep appreciation for difference in human life and activity' (Sneed, 2010, p. 179). Sneed questions liberation theology and by implication critical social theory in that it requires both oppression and a liberating agent. He suggests a more important question is how to engender the valuing of human fulfilment and flourishing. Heron and Reason (1997, p. 282) talk about critical subjectivity: combining reflexivity with critical social theory to generate 'a self-reflexive attention to the ground on which one is standing'. For the newly unemployed Fred (see Case Study), being aware of this ground might mean saying I recognize this is not about me, I continue to have skills and capacities and will explore how these might now be used, I will not continue to blame myself.

Implicit in critical reflection is the expectation that for practitioners it is not enough to work at one level only. In order to achieve change, and from the critical perspective this would mean socially just change (Brookfield, 2005) practitioners need to seek change at a structural level as well as with individuals (Fook, 2002). For Fred this might mean not only working with him about income maintenance or his reaction, but also enabling him to make connections with others in the same or a similar position, reinforcing or exploring the impact of broader change. It might also mean seeking a change in policy or working with communities to generate alternative employment.

This desire for, or expectation of, social change is echoed in the spirituality literature: Ruether, a feminist liberation theologian, identifies the diversity of groups who experience being oppressed in a particular culture and the desirability of such groups working together (2006). She, like Berry (2009), identifies the importance of advocating for the environment and for a socially just approach: 'to repent of power over others and to reclaim power within and power with one another ... This is a vision of life energy that call us all into life-giving community from many strands of tradition, culture and history' (Ruether, 2006, p. 328). From a practitioner perspective, Consedine (in Holloway and Moss, 2010, p. 150) says 'What makes for a holistic spirituality is the recognition that we are all interdependent, that we need to see the divine spark in one another and respect that, and that we need to specifically protect the most vulnerable, the poorest and the most powerless'.

How practitioners do this will vary depending on their role, their work context and on their perceptions of what is possible. It might mean seeking to change an organizational policy or process that doesn't allow for difference. A friend who had to use a wheelchair campaigned to have doors she could open herself instead of having to wait for someone to come. It could mean encouraging an organization to articulate what Huffington et al. (2004) see as the unhelpful assumptions 'beneath the surface'– those internalized at an organizational level. Hearne (2013), for example, identified the pervasive sense of anxiety in an organization and worked with staff to articulate how anxiety was generated and how it could be dealt with more effectively. Alternatively, it might mean contributing to the development of policy change in a particular field of practice or advocating for a service user or community about a specific issue. The 'critical' aspect here provides a limit or balance to what might be perceived as a postmodern sense of anything is possible and equally valued. Support for social justice means advocating for principles that relate to human rights that will underpin practice (Ife, 2008). What this will mean in practice, of course, may be challenging: Brookfield (2005) suggest that we can't know exactly what working from a socially just perspective will mean, until we try it in practice.

Summary

This chapter outlined the four main underlying theories of critical reflection: reflective practice, reflexivity, postmodernism and critical social theory. These reinforce and/or complement each other in providing a stance from which to approach being critically reflective. This includes the capacity to explore emotions, thoughts, reactions and behaviours, assumptions and values; to perceive from a variety of perspectives, to be open to diversity, complexity and uncertainty and to understand the influence of social context and the desirability of working towards socially just change. How spirituality and psychodynamic approaches might relate to these theories has also been briefly explored.

Questions for reflection

- How did you react to the theories identified in the chapter individually and/or collectively? What did you think? How did you feel?
- What did you find appealing and/or what was confusing or irritating?
- How could you see your practice connecting to the theories identified? What might you explore changing in your practice related to the theories identified?

3 Practicing Critical Reflection

While being critically reflective is ideally an attitude to practice, it is also helpful to actively use critical reflection in a focused way to explore specific experiences in a particular context. Given that practitioners have different personalities and preferences and operate in a variety of contexts, it is important to identify a variety of ways in which people can practice critical reflection. These are also useful of course in *learning* how to critically reflect, a skill that develops with practice. This chapter outlines a variety of processes for critically reflecting that can be used on your own, in supervision, in pairs and in groups, within and outside organizations, formally and informally. Chapter 6 considers the use of critical reflection in supervision in more detail.

The importance of establishing the culture or climate of critical reflection was explored at the end of Chapter 1 and it may be helpful to revisit that before starting on any of the critical reflection processes outlined in this chapter. With all of these processes, it does also help to cultivate an attitude of being critically reflective while doing critical reflection. What I mean by this is taking time to create or connect with the inner space in which reflection ideally takes place as well as the outer. Johns (2005a, p. 67) identifies the importance of reflection as a 'way of being' sitting with the 'mystery of experience'. Some would link this to a spiritual sense of seeking meaning. Hick and Bien's (2008, p. 5) ideas about mindfulness, in working with service users, can be equally applied to reflective processes: 'mindfulness is a way of paying attention with empathy, presence, and deep listening that can be cultivated, sustained, and integrated into our work … an innate human capacity to deliberately pay full attention to where we are, to our actual experience and learn from it'. It helps then to slow down, mentally consider the idea of entering a different kind of space of openness to whatever emerges. Some people find it helpful to have a ritual or image or some kind of meditative practice that helps still the mind and let go of other pressing issues (Gardner, 2011, pp. 115–16).

Many possible processes are suggested in this chapter and how to use these is limited only by your creativity. Participants in training sessions often ask how possible it is to critically reflect by yourself. The very idea of being critically reflective affirms the aim of developing the capacity to be critically reflective on your own. However, it can be difficult to fully articulate assumptions and values on your own when they are both implicit and deeply held. The process of having somebody else to ask questions, reflect back and offer or stimulate other ways of thinking can certainly help the process. The processes here can be used or adapted individually, in individual supervision, in 'critical friendships' or 'critical pairs', in supervision groups or in training of various kinds. As Hickson (2013) suggests it is helpful to think about critical reflection as a series of ponds or possibilities, a variety of ways of choosing to reflect that suit you in a particular context at a particular time.

At this stage, I am focusing on how practitioners use critical reflection for themselves, but, of course, these processes could equally be used with service users, groups or communities. I begin with a process of critical reflection with related questions for exploring a specific experience based on the Fook and Gardner (2007) model of critical reflection underpinned by the theoretical approaches outlined in Chapter 2. This is a two stage process and the related questions can of course be used by individuals on their own as well as by supervisors and in groups; it can be used face to face, in writing 'conversations' or journals, or through digital means. An example is worked through in detail later in this chapter to illustrate the process. Other useful examples are Fook's (2000) or Hickson's (2011) experiences. Morley's (2012) article also outlines a specific example from her research demonstrating both stages. The other suggested processes outlined are also influenced by this approach and make clear links between the kinds of questions asked and the movement from exploration to change or action. Depending on the particular process used this may be more implicit or explicit.

Critical reflection: questions and related interactions

Before I explore the specific processes I include some comments about critically reflective questions and interactions. The dilemma in suggesting any questions is that these are then taken to be *the* questions and asked routinely. Ideally, critical reflection is an intuitive and responsive process and questions that arise should be fitting for the person and their particular experience. However, the trouble with not suggesting any questions as examples is that people can find it difficult to work out what kinds of questions to ask. While there are no 'right' or 'wrong' questions, it does seem to help the process to focus on open questions rather than closed, to ask in neutral ways and to remember to ask about feelings as well as thoughts and reactions. To help with this, I have suggested some possible beginning questions at several points in the process (see the figures in this chapter). I have also included questions developed in Southern Health workshops where practitioners identified the kinds of questions or beginnings of questions that were consistently helpful (see the Practice Example 'Questions from Southern Health').

I want to reinforce though that these are only suggestions; it is more important to find the question that seems to work, even if it feels hard to clearly identify it. It is also important to remember that other apparently simple aspects of communication are very effective here: reflecting back to someone what they have said, asking someone to say more about something, paraphrasing or summarizing. Noticing language can help: has the person used words or metaphors that would be illuminating to explore. All of these are useful, as they would be in any other situation, in enabling the person to articulate more clearly for themselves.

Noticing and asking the person to expand on a metaphor can be particularly helpful, providing another way of developing a different perspective. Hickson (2012, p. 836) uses the metaphor of a new coat as a way of exploring how her new assumptions felt: the coat's newness not feeling quite comfortable, needing to stretch it a bit and take up the hem. A workshop participant said she felt like the grit in the oyster, important in making the pearl, but not getting much recognition in the final product. She decided she was sometimes happy to be the grit, but at other times, would like to be the pearl and started to seek acknowledgement for her role.

What generally is not helpful is making suggestions or offering advice: the focus in this process is on the person working things out themselves. Offering advice or suggestions too often comes from your own reaction to their situation. If someone is stuck it can help to *tentatively* offer a possibility: 'I wonder why you did x rather than y' or 'was there any possibility this could relate to …?' Another way to help when someone is stuck is to 'idea storm' possibilities. This is simply having the group – or the supervisor and supervisee- generating possibilities, without evaluating them, to provide more ideas about whatever the person is stuck about – it could be naming feelings, assumptions or possible new ways to act. The person presenting their experience can then use these to react to or to say 'yes, that bit makes sense' or 'none of those really fit, but it makes me think about …'. However, if the person does not connect with a suggestion, it is important to leave it, recognizing that's more likely to be your response than theirs.

Questions from Southern Health

Practice example

Stage one questions
- How do you/did you feel about …? (Noticing and identifying emotions/feelings)
- What does this make you think? (Noticing thoughts)
- What other reasons could there be? (Starting to try to generate ideas about other ways to see situation)
- What did you mean by …? (Noticing language, helping person tease out meaning)
- Where could x be coming from? (Let's idea storm – where might x be coming from?)
- How else might x be experiencing, for example, the conflict, the relationship, the influence of power … ?
- How might x feel?
- What assumptions are being made? – by you and by x?
- How does this work in your situation?
- What room is there for difference?
- How did you feel when … ?
- What if …?
- What else was happening for you?
- How does this relate to other experiences you have had?
- What are your underlying assumptions/thoughts?

Transition questions: towards end of stage one:
- Where are you with this now?
- How would you summarize where you've got to?
- Are you ready to move to stage two?

Stage two questions
- What past assumptions need to be let go?
- Which should be affirmed?
- What new assumptions would be more useful?
- What new assumptions do you want to develop?
- What strategies can you use?
- What could you now do differently?
- What specific strategies could you try?
- What can others suggest – ask for ideas.
- What metaphors might be useful here?

End stage two
Ask if there is any word or phrase that sums up where you have got to and that would reinforce your learning.

Critical reflection processes

Two stage model of critical reflection

As outlined in Chapter 1, Fook and Gardner (2007) defined critical reflection as a theory and a process that 'involves a deeper look at the premises on which thinking, actions and emotions are based. It is critical when connections are made between these assumptions and the social world as a basis for changed action' (Fook and Gardner, 2007, p. 14).

More specifically, critical reflection can be thought of as a way of understanding and engaging with the interconnections between:

- an experience (it helps the process to use a specific experience);
- the emotions, thoughts, reactions and actions related to that experience;
- meaning: what matters about the experience, including related assumptions and values at a fundamental level; and
- the influence of social context and history both individually and collectively with the expectation of the critically reflective process leading to socially just change.

The two stages of critical reflection are:

Stage one: analysis/exploration/deconstruction. At this stage, the emphasis is on:

- exploring how a particular experience is significant to this person;
- identifying hidden or 'taken for granted' theory or assumptions; and
- exploring where the theories or assumptions have originated and whether they fit with the person's preferred values and practices.

Stage two: change/reconstruction. At this stage, the emphasis is on:

- how practice or actions need to change to fit how the person prefers to work to fit with fundamental values; and
- ideas about how to bring about such change: clarification and/or shifts in assumptions or affirming these more actively; suggestions for developing strategies.

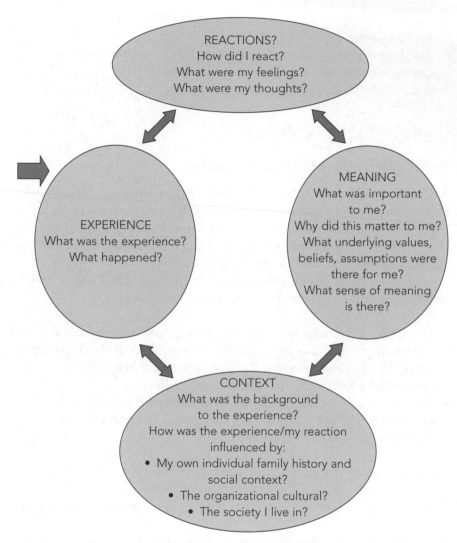

Figure 3.1 Critical reflection stage 1a: exploring my reaction … where was I coming from?

The figures in this chapter represent a way of thinking about the central aspects of critical reflection: experience, reaction, meaning and context. The process of critical reflection here means starting from a specific experience to articulate how you react to the experience and understand its meaning in a particular context. Note that the questions in the figures are only *possible* questions that suggest what might be useful to explore from each area. The arrows indicate the interconnectedness of each aspect and the questions at the bottom of the figure illustrate possible connections for particular individuals.

You can, of course, start exploring at any point, but what is essential is to focus on a particular experience especially when learning the process. Starting with something too broad makes it harder to identify the underlying reactions and meaning. Rather than identifying an issue such as 'my ability to work with angry colleagues' it is more helpful to think about a specific example of where you have found it hard to engage or resolve an issue with a particular angry colleague.

The example on page 57 illustrates how to use these questions or related questions to begin exploring the meaning of this experience (see Figure 3.1). In this example I am working sequentially, starting with the experience, following by reactions, meaning and then context. Helen, the person with the experience, was part of a supervision group that was taking part in a critical reflection training spread over two days. Each person in the group had been asked to bring an experience that they were prepared to explore. Of course, in practice, practitioners are more likely to follow their own internal logic about what sequence to use and it is more a matter of checking that each aspect has been covered.

Finally, it also helps the process for the person with the experience to share a brief written summary of the background to the experience, what the specific experience was and why it is significant – an absolute maximum of one page and preferably less. This begins the process of clarifying and exploring and means that you have to order your thoughts to some degree to write something that will make sense to other people. Particularly for introverts, it is helpful to do this so that you are already processing the experience before you come to the session. I am using Helen's written comments adapted for confidentiality.

Helen

Case study 3.1

Helen's particular experience: I was working in a school as a project officer. I hadn't been in the position for long, about 8 months and the principal who was my supervisor had been very positive and supportive about my work. Then suddenly in a staff meeting, the principal criticized a particular aspect of my project. In the meeting, I felt unable to defend myself and felt physically sick at her judgemental comments. After the meeting, I went home and thought about what she had said and how she had said it. I decided that I should raise this with her the next day, but she was away and when she came back the following week I just let it all go. This experience happened 10 years ago, but it still feels very painful.

Reactions: When Helen was asked more about her reactions to the experience using the kinds of questions shown in Figure 3.1, she responded initially by describing herself as feeling overwhelmed, inadequate and incompetent. She also felt quite angry that the principal had not raised these issues with her in private before raising them in public. Part of her was conscious of thinking that she disagreed, but was not able to come up with an argument to defend herself at the time.

Meaning: When the discussion moved on to where she might have been coming from (what this might have meant for her) Helen named values of respect and loyalty. Teasing these out further she acknowledged that she expected to be respected and seen as a person of worth by a supervisor or manager, which included an assumption that 'if you disagree with someone you talk to them about it privately not publicly'. She realized that she also assumed that a manager would be right, be more powerful and have more authority. These assumptions were to some degree complicated by another assumption about women (the principal was a woman) being emotional and more likely to have inappropriate outbursts of feeling. Overall, the experience meant that she doubted her competence as a practitioner and particularly as a female practitioner.

Context: This exploration connected with thinking about context – the influences from her experience and the broader social context. Helen found this challenging, but said she identified strongly with her Italian Catholic background, seeing both of these as positive influences for her particularly as a child. Although she no longer practiced as a Catholic, she felt she still often reacted as a Catholic. Some aspects of this she felt positive about such as valuing the spiritual, human life and relationships but she acknowledged that her respect for hierarchy was sometimes undermining. In thinking about differences between espoused theory and theory in practice she identified assumptions about gender that were influenced by her Italian background. She also felt the combination of her family and religious background reinforced that conflict was something to be avoided especially with those she perceived as more powerful. In this example, she felt her underlying assumption was 'if I raise this it will make things worse'.

Combining reaction, meaning and context: The discussion then returned to why was this so upsetting, so confronting for Helen, what really mattered to her about it? Her response was that it was painful to acknowledge that she had let herself down by not being prepared to raise this issue directly with her supervisor. In retrospect, she felt that she had made assumptions that had expanded and become more unhelpful in her life: assumptions that she as a woman should not become a manager in case she too reacted emotionally and inappropriately. Being critically reflexive she felt that she had allowed herself to be seen as a person without integrity and competence and that she had taken on board that she did not have these qualities.

Part of the process of critical reflection is identifying and exploring other ways that a particular experience might be seen (see Figure 3.2 on page 60). This is not done to imply somebody 'should' have done things differently. The assumption, influenced by postmodernism, is that any situation can be perceived and reacted to in many different ways and that it will be helpful in the process to consider what some of those other ways might be. When critical reflection is taking place with other people, it is helpful to ask how the other people involved might see this experience – such as the principal in this example. Sometimes people find this almost impossible as their own view is so firmly entrenched. Generating possibilities as a group can assist, that is, simply listing possibilities no matter how unrealistic these may be. Writing these on a whiteboard can also help so that the immediate focus is removed from the person. This seems to free the person from seeing their perception as the only possible one, even if, of course, no one can be sure which variety of perceptions is closest to being accurate.

Helen

Case study 3.1 *continued*

Helen's reactions to these questions: In response to Helen then, people asked, what might the principal be feeling and thinking? Helen found this quite difficult to do, so she asked the others in the group to generate some possibilities. Given that they didn't know the principal, these were all clearly only ideas. What they came up with included:

- she was in a bad mood with everyone because she had had a major argument with her partner over breakfast;
- she had a migraine and couldn't think clearly;
- she forgot that she hadn't raised the issues with Helen;
- she was really irritated by the previous discussion in the staff meeting and spoke without thinking; and
- she was feeling stressed by her workload generally.

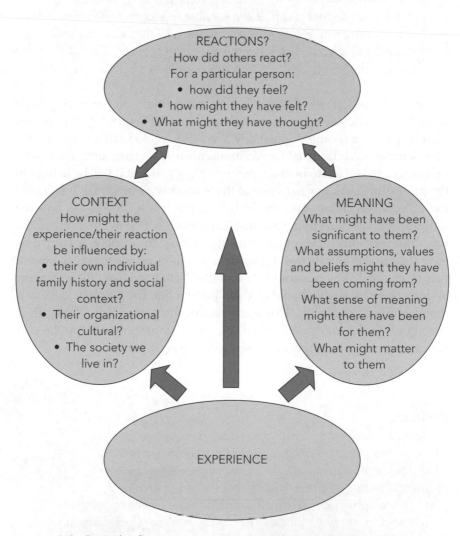

Figure 3.2 Critical reflection stage 1b: what other reactions could there be? Start with a particular person

While Helen could not be sure that any of these applied, she did find it freeing to think that other things might have been happening for the principal, most of which had nothing to do with her. This had the effect of reducing the hierarchical difference between them, so that Helen saw her as another person rather than only in a position of authority. Helen did then remember that the principal was under considerable pressure because of funding cuts recently announced by the government and that the project itself was under threat.

From a critical or social context perspective, the group also asked questions about other experiences related to Helen's identification of cultural influences and assumptions. These included whether Helen had known any men who reacted emotionally in an unhelpful way and whether she had known any women who approach conflict or difference in a calm and constructive way. Helen acknowledged that she did and that this challenged her assumptions about women and women managers particularly. She also acknowledges the variety of people and approaches to conflict both in the Catholic Church and in her Italian community.

Before moving to Stage Two (see Figure 3.3 on page 62), it is useful to ask what the exploration of the experience, the reaction, meaning and context has meant. Is the person reacting differently now? Are there shifts in perceptions, assumptions, understanding of the meaning of the experience? This also clarifies whether the person is ready to move to Stage Two or needs/wants to do more exploring of the experience first. If the person is able to summarize where they are or to identify new assumptions or understanding, it is likely that they are ready to move on. If not, more exploration at Stage One is likely to be needed.

Helen

Helen's experience: At this point, Helen said that she felt quite different about the experience: in retrospect, what was central for her was her not raising this issue with her supervisor. She thought this reflected her own background as well as a more general cultural assumption that you shouldn't question people in authority. This linked to beliefs that she was less powerful, less

Case study 3.1
continued

able to present her views and that if she did it would make the conflict worse. At a more conscious level her espoused theory was the importance of raising issues with people, but her theory in practice was still to withdraw. She was also concerned about her assumptions about gender, feeling that these were undermining both for her and in her attitudes to her daughters. She was keen to start generating ideas about more helpful new assumptions and to think about the implications for changed action.

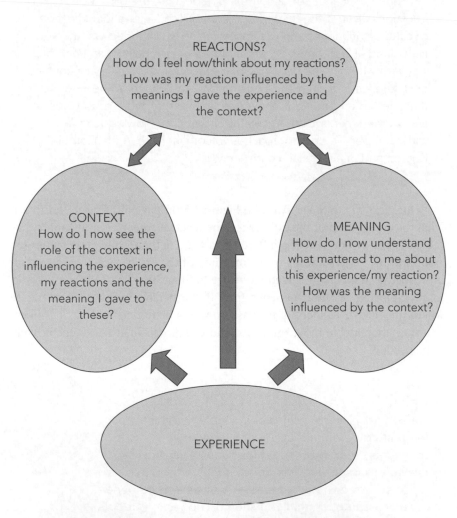

Figure 3.3 Critical reflection stage 1c: new understandings/perceptions – where am I now?

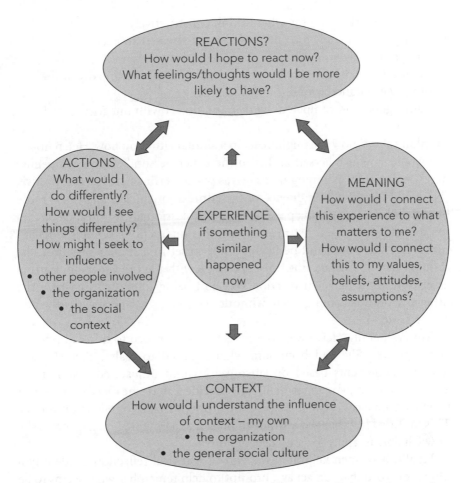

Figure 3.4 Critical reflection stage 2: what difference will this understanding make?

The questions in Figure 3.4 are focused on change. A useful question can be how might I react now if something similar happened?

For Helen, it was more useful to start by asking: where am I now with this experience? She wondered if in some ways she had over-reacted: assumed that she was the problem, that it was her fault, rather than asking: what is happening here? In retrospect, she thought she had internalized a variety of messages that were connected to her own background and experience. She generated some new assumptions:

- This isn't necessarily about me.
- I need to find out what is meant rather than making assumptions.
- Women are equally capable of being good managers.

- I can be assertive and say what I think constructively.
- Managers are people too and may also get stressed and act inappropriately.
- Managers will be affected by what is happening more broadly in the organization and beyond.
- I am a good and competent worker and do act with integrity.

Thinking about how she might react in a similar situation now, Helen hoped she would now ask herself and then the other person 'What is happening here?', rather than assuming that she was wrong. From a critical perspective, she would identify the influence of the context: organizationally and more broadly, what is happening personally and professionally for this person and for me and what does that mean about this interaction? While she recognized that she would still be likely to feel upset in a similar situation, she thought that she would now raise the issue with the other person, putting assertively what her own reaction was and being interested in where the other person was coming from, without assuming their perspectives would be the same.

More generally, Helen was conscious that she needed to think differently about gender. She had been somewhat shocked to realize that she was making judgements based on unconscious and unjustified assumptions about gender and management. She decided that she needed to enlist support from a colleague to help her be more conscious of her assumptions. This included her changed attitude to herself as a potential manager and she now felt able to apply for a management role.

Finally, it is often helpful at the end of a critical reflection to identify a phrase or word that can act as a prompt to help remember what seems to be the key or a key aspect of what has emerged. For Helen, this was the question: 'What is happening here?' She thought this applied equally to her engaging with conflict and power and to questioning assumptions about gender. The question, she thought, would slow her down and encourage thinking rather than just reacting.

Using visual images

Using visual images for critical reflection encourages accessing of different and often unconscious aspects of a person's beliefs and values, feelings and thoughts. Dewey (1934, p. 35) makes a distinction between those experiences that are recognized and those 'experienced but not in such a way that they are composed into *an* experience'. Using something like visual images or writing can help coalesce something elusive into clarity. Field (1983, p. 139) found that it was only when she started paying attention to images that she 'at last became able to use concepts to elucidate everyday experience and so become able to live reflectively rather than blindly'. Wood and Schuck's (2011) book on supervision is a particularly practical resource for using visual images. They document how to use objects like puppets, toys, bricks, stones as well as pictures to encourage creativity in reflection in supervision, but these could equally be used elsewhere. Such resources can be simple and cheaply resourced: toys discarded from children you know or second-hand toys gathered over time; stones and other material found on beaches or in forests. Their value is in how people use them symbolically.

Ways of using visual images vary: an obvious one is to suggest – to yourself or someone else – drawing the particular experience that you want to explore. It is important in doing this to let go the idea of drawing as creating a perfect image. Drawing in this sense is really about visually representing on paper what the experience has meant for you (or the other person). It doesn't matter how clear the image is to anyone else or how aesthetically pleasing it is, what matters is that the process enables expressing something more clearly. In one set of spirituality training, for example, I asked participants to visually represent on paper how they saw their life right now, all of the aspects of their lives that currently engaged them. Looking at this on paper in itself often raised issues for people: the degree of busyness, clarity about why they felt *so* drained of energy, the lack of any space to contemplate and regenerate. I then asked them to use the same image to make the kinds of changes they might want to if they knew they only had one year to live. Again being able to visually represent this, highlighted what people felt about their lives, assumptions they had made about what they needed to be doing, and focused them on what really mattered and the influences that diverted them from this. For more detail about this and related processes see Gardner (2011).

Some practitioners use small figures or models: essentially the kinds of figures that children might use in play and those used in sand play therapy (Wood and Schuck, 2011). These are likely to include figures of people of various sizes and shapes, might include animals, and a variety of more abstract shapes from various substances that can be interpreted at will. These are then used by the person who wants to explore their experience through visual representation of what is happening. In one exercise, a practitioner put together a tiger threatening a mouse in a very small space bounded by high walls and no door. This represented her feelings of being stuck in her workplace and feeling overcome by the pressure to operate in ways that she didn't feel comfortable with. The next step was to think about some kind of change and a question that was useful here was: 'If you could change this to be how you would want it to be how would it be different?' and to encourage the person to physically move the different pieces of her construction. What she did was to simply remove the mouse and place it next to a symbolic tree and leave the tiger no way out of its bounded space. She identified internalized assumptions she had about always 'hanging in there', never giving up, believing that other people were more disadvantaged and that therefore she had to put up with her own situation. Some of these assumptions clearly related to her family expectations, a strongly Protestant work ethic and prevailing cultural values about working hard. Her new assumption was 'I can control the tiger' a metaphor that she used actively to remind herself of her new approach.

Organizations such as St Luke's (www.innovativeresources.org) have developed a wide variety of visual images in the form of cards that can also be used to encourage critical reflection. Some these are purely pictorial, others have a word or phrase that might express a value or belief. People vary in which of these they find useful so it can be helpful to experiment with different kinds. What is helpful about these is again that they represent or generate a way of talking about something that may otherwise be difficult to access. Shadows cards, for example, show images that can be interpreted quite differently: in the same image you might focus on the bleakness of the house or the welcoming light in its window. For more detail on these, visit the website or Gardner (2011).

Of course, there are other ways that people may create visual images or creative ways of exploring a particular experience. Some people prefer to draw or paint more freely to create a different aspect of their experience. Some people might use clay or other material or dance to create an image. Others would use psychodrama and ask people to enact for them a particular experience.

With all of these forms of using visual images, what is important is to use the image to further explore understanding of the experience that it relates to. Sticking with the image is crucial here in unearthing the meaning of it for the particular person and how it connects to the experience they want to understand more deeply. It is useful then to ask questions that are both general questions about the image as well as specific questions related to details, colour, size, shape and so forth. Although I have suggested some questions below, it is important to remember that these are only examples of possible questions. The questions you choose to ask need to suit language you would naturally use and that is appropriate for the person that you are working with.

- So what is the image about? Could you describe the image for me?
- What are the feelings in the image for you? What feelings emerge for you as you look at the image?
- What does the image make you think about?
- What other experience does this connect with?

You might also ask more specific questions or prompt a discussion depending on the particular image:

'What is the significance of the colour of …?' Or simply 'why red?'
'Tell me about this person.'
'How do these parts/people connect?'
'I notice this person is much smaller, what is that about?'

Using writing for critically reflecting

Writing as a way of being critically reflective comes in many forms: journaling, writing creatively, poetry and social media such as blogging. For some people, the process of writing about their experience is helpful in itself in starting the process of engaging with it in a different way. Writing can be a private experience (unless the writer chooses otherwise or it is being used for student assessment), where the writer can feel confident that they are the only person who will have access. It is often useful simply to write without thinking, to have a 'stream of consciousness' approach. In this way, the writer can feel free to say whatever they like without having to think about presenting something more socially acceptable. More direct and honest feelings and thoughts can emerge. Having expressed these feelings and thoughts, the writer can then stand back from the process and contemplate their reactions. Seeing what has been written encourages this process of seeing the experience more dispassionately, being able to consider the strength of the reactions and to start to wonder where these have come from, what they have been influenced by.

Different writers suggest different ways to increase access to what is happening at a less conscious level in such writing. Burchell (2010, p. 396) advocates writing poetry or in a poetic way: 'the significance of seeing a relationship between movement of words and movement of inner self, and how this forms a basis for development of the individual's sense of a "way of being" in their practice world.' Her experience was that writing in a poetic way allowed unformed reactions, feelings and thoughts to surface and become known in a particularly vital way.

Journaling is one of the more frequently used ways of writing for critical reflection. This is simply a process of using writing to clarify or explore a particular experience. Sometimes people think about journaling as a way of having an internal dialogue, but in a way that helps to externalize feelings, thoughts and assumptions. Bolton's (2001) book is a particularly helpful resource for those interested in writing in a critically reflective way. She also suggests creative possibilities for writing. For example, a useful exercise is to first write about an experience from your own perspective; then write about the same experience from the perspective of somebody else who was involved in it. Having completed both of these descriptions, you then write about it from your own perspective for a second time. What often seems to happen in the process is that it becomes clearer what the perspective of the other person might be – and whether or not you know this is the case – having this understanding then shifts the feelings and/or thoughts about how you see the experience yourself. You can of course include in this process more critically reflective questions about assumptions, meaning and the influence of context.

From a more psychodynamic or gestalt perspective, you could also use this exercise to 'talk' with different parts of yourself – see what the conforming part of you might say to the part of you more interested in change. Johnson (1986) calls this working with active imagination and gives an illuminating example of a woman who becomes obsessed with decorating her home. When she dialogues with this part of herself, she discovers a creative side of herself, which at a conscious level she is denying expression.

Journaling can be particularly useful for lone or isolated practitioners who have less opportunity to critically reflect with someone else. Having a series of questions to act as prompts can be helpful here to reduce the possibility of avoiding difficult issues. The kinds of questions that have been identified in this chapter can be used or you could develop your own list of prompting questions that you find helpful as general beginning questions complemented by others that relate to the particular experience you are exploring.

One of the benefits of journaling is that you are left with a written record of your initial reaction and the subsequent changes. This can be useful to look back on and to reflect on whether there are particular issues that emerge as patterns over time.

Other forms of writing for critical reflection are also becoming more popular, particularly social media including social networks, email and blogging (Wright and Bolton, 2012). Any of these can potentially be used for being critically reflective and as more and more people use social media personally, they are also likely to use it professionally. Hickson (2012) interviewed (by email) 10 social workers who used a blog for reflection. Blogs vary, they can be individual and private, shared with a particular group or freely available online. Hickson (2012, p. 43) found 'some blogs that tended to express thoughts and provide description without critical reflection, whilst other blogs provided a depth of reflection that explored assumptions and considered ways to practice in a different way in the future'. There were three main benefits: networking, professional development and self-care, one participant commented:

By using a blog for reflection, I am a better social worker. I take a holistic perspective. It allows me to have catharsis for the sometimes toxic work that I do. It helps me hold on to my humanity when I want to run away from the world and hide. If I am a better human, then I am better neighbour, better spouse, better father, and hopefully a better citizen.

Blogs were also used by physiotherapy students on placement to encourage reflecting on practice (Ladyshewsky and Gardner, 2008). Feedback was positive, students generally found the blog helpful and a flexible, accessible way to maintain communication and develop reflection skills.

Email can also provide scope for reflection. We facilitated a small postgraduate class where participants used a particular experience for critical reflection over a period of 18 months. After an initial face-to-face presentation of experiences and discussion, they used an email exchange to further their exploration of their particular experience and to receive feedback and questions from other students and the facilitators. This enabled the emerging ideas from class to continue to be explored within the culture of critical reflection and led to deepening understanding of issues and recurring patterns. Email, like the blog, also allowed people to respond if and when they wanted to. For some, this felt preferable to the immediacy of face-to-face discussions.

With all of these forms of writing, there are issues of privacy and confidentiality. It is important to be conscious of whether anyone else will see what you have written. If you are a student, for example, you may be conscious of assessment criteria as well as the value of simply writing for your own reflection. Many of the issues for bloggers were similar to those in any group. Some of Hickson's (2012) bloggers mentioned their preference for not being identifiable so that they could speak freely; others who had chosen to give their names were more careful about what they wrote. In Ladyshewsky and Gardner's study (2008) there were similar issues of creating trust as in any group, with some students less willing to communicate in general and participation being influenced by facilitation and due dates for assessment. However, students generally found the blog helpful and a flexible, accessible way to maintain communication.

Meeting to critically reflect

The ways to meet for critical reflection are only limited by imagination and the need to fit with your particular situation. Some practitioners choose to meet face to face in pairs or threes for what might be called 'critical friendship' either in, or separate from, the workplace. I have seen this develop in a number of ways: after a workshop, people might identify somebody else either in their or another workplace that they would like to meet on a regular basis for critical reflection. They might talk about this as a critical lunch or critical coffee and the idea would be to meet on a regular basis probably for about an hour and to take it in turns to talk about a particular experience. In one workplace where all of the members of the team had received critical reflection training, they agreed that they could all call on each other to ask for a session on critical reflection. For this particular team, this more ad hoc approach worked very well, with people feeling free to choose who they felt would be helpful at a particular time.

With the developments of new technologies there are increasingly other ways of meeting: critical reflection by phone, on Skype; or a variety of forms of being linked digitally. All of these can provide ways for practitioners to have a wider variety of people they can critically reflect with at times to suit them. The other advantage of these is that it can provide a critical reflection partner from a completely different perspective: outside the organization or even from a different country.

In some organizations, using critical reflection has become part of the organization's approach to supervision. This will be explored more detail in Chapter 6. Briefly, some organizations have instituted peer or group supervision using critical reflection. They may also or instead include critical reflection in individual supervision. Alternatively, some practitioners choose to have external supervision with a supervisor who uses a critical reflection approach.

With people who are meeting formally to engage in a critical reflection process, it is important to be clear about what process is being used. The process outlined in Fook and Gardner (2007) is one that has been used in many organizations, and adapted to varying degrees to suit the particular context (Fook and Gardner, 2013).

Embedding critical reflection in practice

Being critically reflective probably means that you will use the questions and processes outlined above informally as well as formally and in practice as well as in reflecting on practice in supervision or blogs or journaling.

This might mean, for example, that you include questions in assessments that generate being critically reflective or that you 'research' or evaluate your practice using a critical reflection approach. Using such questions as: 'what other ways can you/we think about this?' would be useful in any assessment, or 'what is the influence of the social context?' These issues will be considered in more detail in the following chapters.

Summary

This chapter focused on how to practice critical reflection processes to develop the capacity to be critically reflective. The 'how' of critical reflection has been thoroughly addressed – including what forms of questions and ways of communicating can help the process. The initial process – the Fook and Gardner (2007) model – has been outlined in detail using a specific example to illustrate the complexity and depth likely in using critical reflection. A wide range of the other processes have also been explored: using visual images, various forms of writing, including social media and meeting with others. The aim is to creatively engage with these to determine what kind of processes for being critically reflective suit you and your context.

- What was your reaction to the process of critically reflecting on Helen's experience? (How did you feel? What did you think?)
- Take an experience of your own and see how you might use the four sets of questions to explore it.
- Which of the processes explored here do you prefer and why?
- How might you develop opportunities to practise these?

Questions for reflection

Critical Reflections
in Organizations

4 Organizational Context

The organizational context is generally named by practitioners as a major influence on and often a major challenge to their capacity to be critically reflective. Practitioners are generally employed in an organization of some kind, funded by government and/or other sources. Even those in private practice have some kind of organization they connect to, even if one person is the manager as well as the practitioner. When practitioners are asked to bring a specific experience to use in training, many bring an experience that relates to how the organization impacts on them and their practice. This might include the organization limiting their capacity to work in ways they see as more effective or creative, being in conflict with organizational values and processes or feeling uncomfortable about specific actions or attitudes of colleagues or managers. It is important to recognize that practice is partly or sometimes largely about how you manage the organization and its dynamic as much as how you carry out the specific professional tasks you are trained for. Frequently, being able to accomplish these professional tasks depends on your skills in negotiating organizational life.

Defining an organization: an entity or constant change?

Those writing about organizations raise questions about how reasonable it is to talk about the organization as a system or entity in this way rather than a complicated and constantly changing mixture of individuals, groups and practices. My sense is that it is helpful to see the organization as both of these. Organizations develop a particular culture or 'feel' that can seem independent of the individuals employed in it and the culture has remarkable staying power over time. Liddell (2003, p. 7) suggests that an organization

> has identifiable boundaries – that is, you can distinguish it from its environment and from other organizations it relates to. The organization has stability in the sense that it is in existence over a period of time, and it maintains relationships with and responds to individuals, groups and organizations in its environment.

On the other hand of course, individuals and groups within organizations can actively seek to change culture. As the productive learning literature suggests, in some organizations at least, there is more recognition of the need to encourage and facilitate the contributions of individuals and groups to organizational life (Boud, Cressey and Docherty, 2006).

Organizational culture and practice

Organizational cultures can take many forms including being constructive, challenging or disabling. Coulshed and Mullender (2001, p. 33) suggest 'organizations are living entities, imbued with the characteristics and inter-relationships of the staff who people them.' My own experience has included such cultures as:

'change should be resisted at all costs';
'we need to be open to whatever will make life better for those we work with';
'only positive events/attitudes are acceptable for discussion';
'we are doing really important work and should support each other to do it as well as possible';
'to feel valued and recognized as a worker you need to convey that you are constantly exhausted and overly busy'; and
'the work we do is more important/more stressful than any other organization.

Some of these are easier to work with than others and you may have experienced quite different ones. Each prevailing attitude has a significant influence on workers individually and collectively within the organization and on relationships with those in other organizations. The culture that implies that to be valued you must be or look exhausted and busy will obviously add to the stress already experienced by workers.

Dina's experience initially seemed very simple: she was feeling embarrassed about leaving work on time. In her previous organization, staff had been encouraged to manage their workload as nurses within set working hours, except in emergencies. Dina had organized other aspects of her life around this: childcare and playing netball. She thought this meant she used her time at work well and managed life better overall. In this

Practice example

organization, however, what was valued was staying late, being or at least talking about feeling stressed and busy. When she left on time she felt she was violating the group culture and perceived as less committed to her role. Reflecting critically on her experience reinforced her desire to contribute to changing the culture rather than becoming part of it.

Practice is constantly influenced by organizational policies and processes both formal and informal, all of which have assumptions like these embedded in them. A simple example that causes tension in many organizations is the policy on access to cars for visiting service users or communities: first, is it possible? or does the organization take the view that service users and community members should demonstrate their motivation by coming to the organization? If the organization, on the other hand, supports visiting service users in their homes or communities, how easy is it for workers to access cars? Do some staff have easier access than others; are cars available after hours or only nine to five, do staff need to get permission to use cars or is their professional judgement sufficient? What are the informal expectations about car use? What are the attitudes to being back later than expected? Responses to all of these reflect individual and organization assumptions. For example, the expectation that service users should demonstrate motivation by coming to the organization implies that this generates the same challenges for all service users. Clearly, this is not the case, not all service users have cars, access to public transport varies, some service users will have to bring children with them or find ways to have them cared for. I have worked in organizations where there was minimal funding for cars, so the assumption was that all the work took place at the organization; in others the assumption was that workers must go out, to experience for themselves the context for the individual or community they were working with. How organizations operate and the implicit assumptions in policies and processes has a direct effect on practice.

Issues in organizational life

The nature of organizational life will also be influenced by the broader social, economic and political context. Sturgeon (2010, p. 1049) identifies the pressure on senior managers and organizations to 'simultaneously compete in a new market like environment, meet a variety of centrally dictated targets and standards, and demonstrate that they can cooperate with other organizations in the healthcare system'. He suggests 'the increasingly market-driven and bureaucratic approach to healthcare in the National Health Service in England has resulted in a system in which measurement and outcome are considered the most important indicator of quality; and yet, in the case of the mid Staffordshire National Health Service foundation trust, this criterion not only failed to ensure the delivery of high quality care, but actively contributed to its prevention'. Huffington et al. (2004) identify related challenges such as the rapid development of information technologies, expectations of competition across globalized markets, changing social and cultural patterns, emphasis on consumer rights and the emergence of a contract culture. These they suggest contrast with an 'an emphasis on innovation and creation' that 'rubs up against the pressure on delivery and results'. These changes have been exacerbated by global financial issues that provide a backdrop to the pressures experienced by practitioners within organizational contexts.

More specifically, these particular issues continue to be emphasized in practitioners' experiences:

Change and uncertainty

Change and uncertainty are inevitable and continuing aspects of organizational life. They are managed better, both by organizations and individuals, when acknowledged and discussed and seen as offering opportunities as well as challenges. Baldwin (2004, p.48) suggests that 'the attempt to manage out uncertainty is to destroy the potential opportunities for dynamic creativity present in managing uncertainty'.

Such change can be externally driven, either in the immediate context of the organization's community, funding and relationships or more generally in the broader political and social environment. Individuals and organizations may react differently depending on where the change has come from, who has initiated it and how. 'Change that has its origin in the environment cannot, as it were, be "wished" away ... although ... for a time (it) can be denied' according to Obholzer and Miller (2004, p. 38), whereas 'Change that is internally generated, by contrast, can be "hived off" ... the institutional equivalent of the body walling off an infection'. They also suggest that the unconscious dynamics of family life may emerge again in response for individuals to change and uncertainty especially if the organization doesn't acknowledge reactions to change.

The current focus on risk is often a way of seeking to manage change and particularly uncertainty. In an environment dominated by the possibility of things going wrong nationally and internationally, individuals and to some extent organizations feel they have less control. Giddens (1999, p. 24) says risk 'is the mobilising dynamic of a society bent on change' and that our consciousness of this is related to having less control of life in general. This is partly, he suggests, because risk is now manufactured to some degree – what we do to nature as well as what nature does to us. Risk is not necessarily negative, risk can generate energy and is an inevitable aspect of change. However, the reaction to what feels like too much risk can be to maximize what can be controlled and to try to guess what might go wrong so that it can be prevented. Organizations advertise now for risk managers whose role it is to plan to avoid potentially damaging situations. The danger can be that so much time and energy goes into this that we lose the capacity to react actively and creatively when something unpredictable does happen. This happens on a small as well as larger scale.

Participants in workshops frequently give examples related to risk. One felt immobilized by her healthcare organization's policy that only those trained to do so could touch patients and move them physically. When faced with a patient clearly about to fall out of bed, she was torn between the need to respond to the person's vulnerability and the organizational rules. Another gave an example of the forms she would need to fill in to take a small group of older people outside their residential facility; it was so daunting she decided it was just too hard. Obviously safety is important and related to the ethics of care, but needs to be balanced with other aspects of caring for a person.

Issues related to change and uncertainty will be explored in more detail in Chapter 8.

Siloed nature of organizational life

Another issue related to funding is that many organizations are only funded for quite narrowly defined fields of practice: the opposite to a holistic approach to practice. An organization might have a drug and alcohol or housing focus, or work with families with a particular kind of disability or those over or under a certain age. Any of these ways of creating categories means the organization expects to work on only that aspect of potential issues for service users. In practice of course, service users often experience a range of interconnecting issues. This then becomes another source of frustration for practitioners who can see more effectiveness in engaging with an individual or family across all or most of their issues, rather than advising them to approach a series of other organizations as well. This partly of course reflects the prevailing culture and context and will depend on the particular organization.

Some organizations are seeking to challenge this way of working either by working more collaboratively across organizations and/or by encouraging more interdisciplinary practice. Both of these will be explored in more detail in Chapter 9 but briefly, these approaches start with thinking how might this work best for the consumer.

> The Western Cluster staff, a mixture of disciplines working in mental health (Gardner, 2013), were particularly able to articulate this dilemma using the metaphor of an iceberg. They suggested that often there was a tension between managers who really wanted to focus on what was visible above the water, what they called the ice, whereas they also wanted to explore the berg: what was not visible. Their assumption was that they needed to understand the underlying cause or the underlying values or meaning that was influencing the particular symptoms of mental illness and to work holistically with all of the issues facing their service users. Managers were often experiencing pressure from more senior managers and funding bodies to demonstrate outcomes in the specific areas funded.

Practice example

Espoused values versus values in action

This dichotomy is one identified by Schön in his writing about reflective practice and discussed in relation to individuals in Chapter 2. It can become even more complex in thinking about life in an organization. The worker's own, often unconscious, assumptions and values, can become entangled with the organization's implicit expectations in ways that undermine or conflict with the espoused values of both. Savaya, Gardner and Stange (2011) write about the experience of Maya, who worked with a mother of children in care who had requested that two of her children return to live with her because of her changed circumstances. Maya initially supports this mother's view that her children should be returned to her care. What becomes clear is that although her espoused theory was to be an 'agent of change' supporting her service user, her theory in action was to be loyal and conform to the norms of the organizational culture, which reduced or eroded her capacity to advocate for her service user. Organizations, of course, or work teams, expect this kind of loyalty – often implicitly, which gives rise to such dilemmas. An organization might also have espoused theory in contradiction to its values in action: for example, an espoused belief that people can change versus reluctance to take risks in practice.

This is often a contradiction that workers experience as frustrating. Organizations have mission statements that identify what they ideally would like to be doing or their preferred philosophy – their espoused values. These are often – for good reasons – broad, general and inspirational. For many staff, this ideal is what appealed to them about the organization initially. It can be quite disillusioning then to find that there is a significant difference between the theory of how the organization operates and its practice. This is not to suggest that organizations should not name the ideal: rather that it is helpful to also name the challenge of trying to live up to it.

This often connects to the emphasis on outcomes as opposed to processes: organizations are increasingly expected by their funding bodies to provide clear evidence about their effectiveness and of course this is a reasonable expectation in terms of justifying public spending. It is obviously easier to do this by providing statistical data about what specific tasks and objectives have been achieved or how many services have been provided. However, this is often a source of frustration for professional practitioners who identify as more difficult goals those that are harder to define and evaluate. Establishing relationships with service users is the initial challenge for many, given their past experience and the complexity of their issues. In New Zealand, the absence of compassion in healthcare led to a campaign to mandate for its inclusion in the New Zealand Code of Patient Rights as a specific, measurable outcome. The campaign was unsuccessful partly on the basis that it is impossible to legally require people to feel compassion and to measure it. As Paterson (2011, p. 21) says: 'I may be deeply touched by the small act of a doctor touching my arm before a painful procedure; how would I feel if I knew that protocol 3.2 required this act?'

> **Practice example**
>
> Sam's organization, which worked with people with a mental illness, had a funding agreement that each service user could have a maximum of 12 sessions. In that time, the expectation was that service users would show significant progress in relation to housing and employment and/or finding meaningful activity. Sam felt very frustrated that what he felt was significant progress in working with a service user called Frank was not recognized in this agreement. Frank had had 15 years of conflict with mental health services and had been labelled difficult and impossible to work with. As a result of this Sam had assumed that he needed to start

by building a relationship with Frank before suggesting work on specific goals. He had by session 11 established a positive relationship: where Frank described as Sam being 'all right': Sam's supervisor who had previously worked with Frank acknowledged the significance of this, but such gains had no place for recognition in the organization's evaluation processes.

Complexities of power

Power is a complex issue in organizations. It often feels to practitioners that those who are powerful are those more senior in the organization and, of course, that is often the case. However, power is exercised in many ways: workers can also be powerful because of their passion and commitment to the organization and its ideals and/or to the service users and communities they engage with. Some exert power simply by being stubborn; others by the depth of their skills or the length of their experience in the organization or the field of practice; others through building collegial relationships and alliances. Supervisors and managers in critical reflection training often testify to this complexity: and how often they feel powerless. Sometimes this relates to broader policy and funding issues, but frequently also to how difficult they find it to get practitioners to do what they as managers think is best when that view is not shared by practitioners. All of these factors apply to working across organizations as well.

Paula worked as a psychologist in a small community-based organization funded by a government department. She met with a family, where the parents and their 14 year old were in conflict, and Julie, the government department representative. Paula was aware from previous contact that Julie wanted to criticize her approach, but was uncomfortable with conflict. What surprised Paula – and what she wanted to explore about the meeting – was how powerful she felt in her role as a worker. Although, in theory, Julie had more power as the representative of the funding body, Paula felt that she had significantly more knowledge and experience that showed in her comfort in raising challenging issues with the

Practice example

family. She became aware of her own sense of authority and power and that Julie found her threatening. This shifted her assumptions about power from: 'I don't have any power' to 'I am powerful and can be positively authoritative given my experience and skills'.

The emotional life of organizations

Implicit in much of the above is the idea of an organization as an entity generating its own culture and by implication its own emotions. Armstrong (2004, p. 11) suggests that '(E)very organization is an emotion place … because it is a human invention, serving human purposes and dependent on human beings to function' and because of that 'alertness to the emotional undertow of organizational life can be a powerful source of information for managers and leaders in enlarging understanding, reviewing performance, foreseeing challenges and opportunities and guiding decision and action'. Such variations in emotion are more likely at times of change and uncertainty, during and after traumatic events, either internally or externally. 'Organizational dynamics are constructed from the interaction between emotions, (such as envy, guilt, anxiety and emotions that are avoided or ignored), and power that create the social and political context within which both learning and organizing can take place' (Vince, 2001, p. 1326). For some people, the emotions experienced in other past and current areas of life such as family or previous work experience can be sparked in times of stress, 'particularly if the institution is led and managed in such a way as to turn a blind eye to such issues' (Obholzer and Miller, 2004, p. 39).

Identifying the emotions that an organization is experiencing overall can therefore help with this, simply inviting those involved to name what is happening. Hearne (2013) used critically reflective processes to research the role that anxiety was playing in her organization and how critical reflection could be used to influence this. A group of staff met four times and used a metaphor of 'the pink elephant in the room' to name those issues like anxiety not acknowledged in the organization.

The participants used the critical reflection process to challenge the assumptions underlying the theory of anxiety in session one. This resulted in changes to views of anxiety, conflict and changed behaviour. This can be understood as a collective process which promoted organizational learning. (Hearne, 2013, p. 137)

What is key from a critically reflective perspective is recognizing first the multiple kinds of emotion and that 'any model of emotions mobilized should be subject to critical analysis, and emotions should not be seen as asocial or "outside" of politics' (Sawn and Bailey, 2004, p. 123).

Organizational culture of critical reflection

Ideally, being critically reflective needs to become part of the general organizational culture rather than something that particular individuals or groups do. As Reynolds and Vince (2004, pp. 3–4) argue, managers are likely to say reflection is important: 'However, the implementation of processes for reflection, especially those that move beyond individuals' responsibility to ensure that reflection happens, remains a poorly developed aspect of organizational experience and action.' They work from a critical perspective, that is, 'reflection should draw on ideas and analytical perspectives which are capable of deconstructing these (managers and professionals) interests and political processes'. Creating a culture of critical reflection can happen in a variety of ways given that the aim is to have being critically reflective permeate through the organization. It does, however, help the process to have endorsement by management either of this general approach or of specific strategies that can be used to embed critical reflection in the organization. This is complicated by differing levels of understanding of critical reflection. A manager might see critical reflection as simply a supervision tool, rather than understanding that being critically reflective might have implications for the organization as a whole, including that staff might feel more confident to challenge existing practices. From her interviews with social workers, Hickson (2013, pp. 194–5) found that learning to be reflective is influenced by a range of organizational factors including:

> the nature of how people work together, the workplace culture in relation to learning and whether the organization values and encourages reflective supervision. However, it was evident that some organizations and their structures and cultures act to limit reflective approaches. The evidence is there that, for social workers, learning to be reflective in organizations is influenced by whether the organizational culture promotes sharing of knowledge and power and whether they feel like they have a voice and can express their views.

Some organizations have had a more formal and concerted approach to implementing critical reflection (Gardner and Taalman, 2013; Thomson, 2013) with varying levels of success. In another organization a large, hierarchical, government department, the senior managers had engaged in the process of critical reflection and decided to implement training for frontline workers and their managers. Both sets of workers embraced critical reflection enthusiastically and as a result of using critical reflection in supervision, the front line workers and their managers began to seek various kinds of changes in the organization. The next line up managers (the middle managers), who had not been involved in either the initial discussions or training, were surprised and unimpressed by this. They effectively blocked most of the suggested changes, with a resulting loss of morale. Eventually, one of the senior managers wanted to evaluate the use of critical reflection and realized what was happening and arranged training for the middle managers, which shifted their responses.

At another organization, a bottom-up approach was successful. A worker had become interested in critical reflection as part of his university training as a social worker. After he had been working for some time in an organization, he asked his supervisor whether she was interested in using critical reflection as a part of their supervision. The supervisor decided to attend a critical reflection workshop and became convinced that this would fit the organization's general philosophy. They then agreed to trial this with a supervision group for their team, using a combination of material from the training. The team was initially reluctant to move to a group model, so a compromise was agreed of some individual supervision and regular group sessions. As this team became convinced about the value of critical reflection in group supervision, others in the organization became interested too. Eventually, training in critical reflection was held in the organization and a series of peer supervision groups established. A third organization wanted to use critical reflection not only in supervision, but as how they approached their work in general. When a new policy or process issue emerged, for example, or when they were confronted with major change, they used this approach in staff meetings to engage with what this might mean and how they might respond.

However, often practitioners wrestle with how to maintain a critically reflective stance in an organization with different priorities. Some do successfully generate processes or strategies that enable them to feel supported in being critically reflective within the organization. Some possible processes were discussed in Chapter 3 and supervision strategies will be discussed in the Chapter 6. What is important here is to note that organizational issues and the organizational context need to be acknowledged as part of what affects an individual practitioner and their capacity to reflect in any organization.

Examples: using critical reflection to explore organizational context

The following examples demonstrate how critical reflection can be used in exploring the influence of organizational context: first an individual engaging with organizational issues and second, how a team used critical reflection training to explore common themes in their experience of their practice in an organization working with people who had been sexually abused.

David's experience

Case study 4.1

An individual worker using critical reflection to engage with organizational issues.

Background: I am a speech therapist in a large rural health service and was supervising a specific student who I will call Vicky, who just didn't seem to be getting what she was supposed to be doing. I had started a procedure with a patient with Vicky observing. I was called to the phone and when I came back Vicky had kept going with the procedure in a way potentially damaging for the patient. I talked to her about my concerns and then to Jane who coordinates the students and asked her to give Vicky feedback that she was in danger of failing her placement. At the next two coordinator meetings Jane said that Vicky had taken the feedback well and strategies were in place.

Specific experience: I hadn't seen any real change in Vicky's work and so said she might fail at the next meeting. It became clear that Jane had painted the problems in a fairly rosy light as Vicky had said she didn't like negative feedback. I felt really angry with Jane as she also hadn't let the university know there were problems with the placement and now wanted someone else to do that.

Significance: Quality of work is really important to me, what I'd call clinical excellence, it seems that this is being compromised constantly in the organization and this is just yet another example.

Stage one

When David was asked more about his anger, he said his underlying values were being 'trampled on': particularly his desire to provide the best possible care. Eventually, he unearthed his underlying assumption that part of providing the best care is facing what you aren't doing well so that you can do it better. He also felt his clinical experience was being ignored and so he felt devalued. It became clear his frustrations were partly about the student's quality of work, but really more about Jane not validating and responding to his concern.

When asked again so what really most bothered him about this, David said he felt disillusioned about the team culture: the differences between espoused theory and theory in practice. When he thought about this in relation to the team and its relationship to the organization he started to generate more examples:

- patients come first vs the organizational rules and expectations come first;
- clinical excellence is the primary goal vs doing well in the organization is the primary goal: getting on the fast track to management.
- Feedback is more important than personal discomfort vs looking good/making things look all right is more important.

This raised the question for David: how do I survive in an organizational culture that feels contrary to my beliefs and ways of doing things. How do I not succumb to the pressure to conform or more likely how do I not get disillusioned and embittered by all this?

This seemed a point of transition to Stage two and when David was asked so where are you now? He responded that he was clearer about why this experience bothered him, the real issue was the organization culture and how to engage with that – or whether he needed to leave.

Stage two

At this stage, David wanted to affirm his original assumptions about clinical excellence, but recognized from a postmodern perspective, he was generating unhelpful binaries. His new assumptions were:

- I can't assume everyone will have the same values and expectations as me, but I can affirm my own.

- Clinical expertise should override seniority in clinical issues: I can use my knowledge, experience and skills to argue for high quality practice.
- I need to recognize my emotions more and when I am exhausting myself with being angry.

He conceded that he enjoyed supervision and mentoring of students and staff and could see how to develop opportunities to affirm quality of practice. At this point, he acknowledged that he partly felt stuck for personal reasons, that the job suited his family, so he also had to make compromises. With the group he generated some strategies about how he could influence the team and organizational culture: suggesting a critical reflection group for students and a separate one for interested staff, individual mentoring, being prepared to ask the 'difficult' questions with managers and in staff meetings. He decided he would call himself 'the quality man' (from a local advertisement) as a way of reinforcing the learning from the session and reminding himself to see the funny side where possible, and to stand back to see the bigger picture.

Megan's and Kate's experiences

Case study 4.2

An organization offering sexual abuse counselling requested critical reflection training for one of their teams. Each person in the group of eight brought a specific experience and as we worked on these common themes began to emerge. The session ended with a discussion about the organization's culture and how critical reflection might be used to engage with and change the culture. I have summarized two of the individual experiences below, then explored their connections to the common themes and the organization culture.

Megan had been to a meeting with community organizations and the police about service coordination and made a critical comment about the police not following the current legislation as closely as they should. One of the police reacted negatively commenting they did what they could given their workloads. She felt misunderstood, put in the position of opposition, which she acknowledged could be how she was perceived generally. She felt torn between wanting to convey an attitude of respect reflecting her assumptions: we are all on the same side, I am a reasonable person, but, on the other hand, her value: truth must prevail, there is one truth. As she explored this further, she recognized reluctantly the potential in herself to push a view in a way that wouldn't allow the other person to express their perspective. She decided she needed to balance the 'truth' with a more postmodern openness in a new assumption: there are many ways to see/experience any situation combined with my way may be the right way but I need to express that respectfully.

Kate's first stage focused on a family experience where she challenged her new sister-in-law who commented they told me you were the over the top one in the family. She had felt 'put back in her box' by this, because she had seen herself as the family peacemaker rather than the troublemaker. As she reflected, she realized that she had unconsciously decided to stop being the active peacemaker, but that she was left with feelings of guilt and anger. It was taking more energy not to be the peacemaker than to take on the role. She suddenly realized that this was also how she felt at work: that she didn't want to be seen as 'over the top' so she repressed her preference for actively seeking to resolve conflict. She thought that her assumption: it's better to tackle conflict directly and manage/resolve it was in tension with the organization culture of let's hope that the conflict/differences will resolve themselves.

Next the group contributed ideas about what they saw as common issues arising from the individual experiences:

- How you communicate negative/difficult messages/ disagreements?
- Seeing complexity can make it more difficult to act/be clear about what's right.
- Where is the place of anger? Is it always destructive?
- Frustration of sexual abuse work, people not asserting themselves.
- What about passion/conviction about what we are doing?
- How do we sustain ourselves in believing we can change things when so much of what we do is about despair?

When they reflected as a team on the cumulative impact of their specific experiences, they felt overwhelmed by the difficulty of their work, how hard it was to live up to their organization's overall aims: to prevent sexual abuse by changing the culture of the society in which they lived. One participant then pointed out that from a critical social theory perspective they *were* making a difference with individuals and families. They were changing internalized views about the acceptability of abuse and that this in itself would change the culture over time. Another reminded the group of the various workshops and school visits they did that also aimed to change culture. The group reflected how influenced they were by external and internal expectations that success could only be measured by reduced rates of sexual abuse.

The group then turned to some of the specific themes: particularly the tension between identifying truth or being right with allowing for other points of view. They reflected that because there is a an obvious 'right' or 'truth' in this work that sexual abuse is not acceptable, having to constantly assert this in the community can predispose workers to assume there is always *the* truth or *the* right way. Their awareness of the lack of power of service users meant they felt they needed to present their views powerfully in opposition if necessary. Thinking back to her example about the police, Megan could see that her assumption was you are with us – and therefore agree with everything I say – or you are against us. Kate suggested that this oppositional or binary way of thinking also influenced her feeling about raising issues within the organization: we have to agree so that we are a coherent group to combat the different views outside the organization. This meant that the organization did not allow the exploration of internal organizational conflict: the assumption was disagreement is dangerous.

The group then questioned: how can we live with a greater complexity about our work and how we do it? Megan's new assumption was discussed again, partly because Kate had also resonated with it: there are many ways to see/experience any situation combined with my way may the right way but I need to express that respectfully. This led to thinking about strategies that could help with this: recognizing emotions and assumptions, learning to stop and wait, allowing for complexity, thinking how to say what needed to be said, being assertive rather than aggressive or passive. What struck the team was how much what they had said about how they expressed difference reflected the struggles in their service users' experience and so how important it was to model assertive communication for service users as well. They agreed the complexity of these issues would remain challenging, but decided to use critical reflection in a peer supervision group as a way of continuing to develop their awareness and processes.

Summary

Practitioners are often surprised by how much the organizational context influences their practice. Understanding the organization as an entity as well as the staff within it is a key aspect of being able to practice effectively. Critical reflection enables practitioners to recognize the dynamics of organizations and the influence of context, the challenges of living with uncertainty and change, issues of structure, power and emotions. Making these conscious enables practitioners to see how their own emotions, reactions, assumptions and values interact with those of the organization and how to develop strategies to manage ensuing issues effectively.

Questions for reflection

- How does your organizational context affect your practice? What is your reaction – how do you feel, what do you think, what do you do?
- What are the assumptions and values that are:
  - Explicit in your organization's mission/vision statement?
  - Implicit in how your organization operates?
  - Where there are differences, what tensions/challenges does this generate for you and/or your team?
  - What assumptions are implicit in your reactions?

Critical Reflection and
Organizational Learning

Being critically reflective encourages an attitude of identifying what is of
value, what works and what doesn't in practice and in organizational life
more generally. Individuals and groups engaging with their experiences
identify not only what they might want to change in their own attitudes or
practice, but also what wider changes, including organizational changes are
desirable. This raises questions about how the organization can learn from
these reflections: how can individuals or groups influence organizational
culture or processes. Is it enough that individuals or groups change or seek
change in their own practice? Will this in itself bring about organizational
change? Does this individual learning need an organizational culture of
learning to be influential? Or alternatively, does an organization need its
own broader reflective processes and structures? What difference does it or
might it make if an organization formally endorses or uses a critically reflective approach? Does it or would it make it easier to be critically reflective if
the organizational culture embodies the attitudes and concepts of organizational learning? This chapter engages with these questions initially by
exploring related literature on organizational learning. This is followed by
identifying ways that individuals, groups and organizations can more
consciously use critical reflection to foster being critically reflective at an
organizational level. These might be described also as developing a researching or evaluating attitude to organizational learning and to practice more
specifically.

How does change happen in organizations?

The questions of how change comes about in organizational practice reflect
the broader issues raised in thinking about transformational learning. Like
critical reflection, transformational learning has also developed from a
number of philosophical and theoretical underpinnings. Transformational
learning 'suggests not only change in *what* we know or are able to do but also
a dramatic shift in *how* we come to know and we understand ourselves in
relation to the broader world' (Dirks, 2012, p. 116). There are differences in

transformational learning approaches about emphasis: for example, whether the emphasis should be on the self or the 'world outside the self and the individual's position in that world rather than on the self' (Cranton and Taylor, 2012, p. 9). They advocate moving beyond such perceived differences to a more unified view that change will happen in diverse ways in different contexts and involve both the individual and their social environment. Critical reflection in combining critical social theory with other perspectives demonstrates this; it allows for individuals to explore the assumptions and values embedded in the social context they have also internalized. This moves beyond the either/or of individual/social context or individual/ organization to seeing how they are interconnected. Critical reflection also fosters transformative learning by starting where the learner is, from their own experience of assumptions and values (Mezirow, 2012).

Thinking about how organizations learn or how learning happens in organizations raises again the question identified in Chapter 4: is it reasonable to think about an organization as a separate entity or is it a collection of individuals and groups engaging in constant activity and change? To create a culture of openness to learning and to change, again it is helpful to move beyond dualities, to think about organizations in both ways. The organization is an entity with formally endorsed structures and its own culture with attitudes that influence learning. Individuals are able to use reflections on practice to generate new possibilities or reinforce effective practice and in turn to influence organizational change. Schatzki (2006, p. 1868) supports this view, suggesting that organizations have collective and cultural memories 'accumulated knowledge about the organization's past and that passed on sub-set of this knowledge that stabilizes a collective identity for members'.

Culture and learning in organizations

Ideas about learning and work or workplace learning vary, as Scheeres et al. (2010, p. 13) say 'learning discourses pervade contemporary workplace and organizational literature'. Their view is that learning is an integral aspect of work and needs therefore to be formally embedded in 'integrated development practices'. These are not part of training programmes, but rather part of how work is done and supervised by managers not trainers. They suggest key questions relate to how learning is regarded in organizations. Some writers have seen the organization as the focus for learning in 'learning organizations', which Brown and Harvey (2006, p. 404) suggest have 'the involvement of all employees – management, non-management, professional, line functions, staff and so forth – in continuous self-directed learning that will lead toward positive change and growth in the individual, team and organization'. Implied in this, is that all individuals will be equally committed to organizational learning, but as Boud and Solomon (2003) found political and identity factors such as position, recognition and power in the workgroup or organization influence whether individuals engage in learning and whether it is perceived positively to be a learner. Certainly, the organizational culture influences how learning is seen and what is possible.

How learning is defined and experienced

Learning in an organization is complex, as Gould (2004, p. 2) suggests and he reinforces that learning happens at many levels:

> the learning experience is more pervasive and distributed than that delivered through a specific, designated training or education event; learning incorporates the broad dynamics of adaptation, change and environmental alignment of organizations takes place across multiple levels within an organization, and involves the construction and reconstruction of meaning and world views within the organization.

This construction and reconstruction of meaning relates to the use of reflection: identifying the assumptions embedded in the culture individually and collectively and being able to change these as needed. Much of this resonates with how critical reflection will be explored in the next chapter: the value of being critically reflective informally as well as in a variety of activities across the organization including individual and group supervision. These activities also enable identifying assumptions in organizational culture that are supporting or undermining practice. Research affirms that assumptions about learning vary depending on organizational culture: Scheeres et al. (2010), for example, found the culture in one organization, a large manufacturing company, fostered seeing learning as part of on the job practice for everyone; in another, an academic environment, learning was seen as 'what students' do, not part of the broader work culture.

Scheeres et al. (2010, p. 19) identify the UNESCO Committee Report 'Learning: the Treasure Within' (1996) as an important development in thinking about learning more broadly. The Committee identified four types of learning that support a critically reflective approach to learning in organizations. They suggest that learning is about *knowing*: knowledge acquisition, but also 'learning to learn, so as to benefit from opportunities education provides throughout life'; *doing*: 'being able to put the knowledge into practice in a variety of situations, adapting as needed'; learning to *be*: being able to act with 'greater autonomy, judgment and personal responsibility', recognizing that learning takes place in a social context, with particular cultural meaning and fourth learning to live and work together in a 'spirit of respect for the values of pluralism, mutual understanding and peace'. This framework is congruent with being critically reflective: understanding the importance of knowing, doing and being and how these are influenced by social context and values.

Can learning change organizational culture?

Other literature also suggests the value of people working in groups or teams to encourage learning. Wenger (2000) considers that for organizations to be successful they need to come to grips with the social nature of learning, as suggested in critical reflection, to understand how learning is influenced by our own and the general context and history: 'learning is an interplay between social competence and personal experience'. Wenger also suggests a more holistic approach, that 'Learning combines personal transformation with the evolution of social structures' (Wenger, 2000, p. 227). In his view what is important is social learning structures or 'communities of practice', which involve mutual engagement and 'an opportunity to negotiate competence through an experience of direct participation' (Wenger, 2000, p. 229). However, he also points out that all communities can be 'cradles of the human spirit, but they can also be its cages' and that it is important to articulate for each community its learning energy, mutuality and sense of social capital and its repertoire: the degree of self-awareness (Wenger, 2000, p. 230). Li et al. (2009) reviewed experiences of communities of practice. They found a tension between Wenger's emphasis on self-empowerment and professional development and the organization's view of communities of practice as a management tool encouraging competitiveness. However, much of Wenger's view of communities of practice fits with creating critically reflective groups and opportunities based on a culture of critical acceptance. The challenge, as he suggests, is how to convey the learning from the community of practice to the organization more generally.

As a result of my own interest in how a critically reflective way of being can influence organizational practice I interviewed 20 professionals who had participated in critical reflection workshops at least six months previously (Gardner, 2007). The interview questions related to what, if anything, had changed in the organization as a result of the participant's involvement in the workshop. Of the 20 participants, 14 identified specific changes in their own behaviour such as more awareness of self and its impact on practice and openness in relationships; 13 were using critical reflection processes in their practice with a greater awareness of underlying assumptions and values. One said that her experience 'encapsulated a moment in time which gives a practice that can be used in other circumstances'. About half the group could identify some kind of change in the culture, such as a 'subtle change in the atmosphere of the team – a good team work feeling'. Six of the 20 believed that their own individual change was changing the organization and nine were using critical reflection in ways they thought contributed to change in the organization.

However, a significant minority (6 of the 20) considered that it wasn't possible for them to actively seek change without more formal organizational support. Similarly, comments from some of the participants in the Pastoral Care Networks Project said that while they had changed individually, it was difficult to get the organization to recognize and validate the change (Gardner and Nolan, 2009). Although the palliative care philosophy theoretically included spirituality, in practice, healthcare managers tended to see this as a specialized rather than a generic role. After the training, practitioners were keen to work in a more holistic way, including spirituality in their practice where appropriate and referring to the specialist pastoral care worker if not. Participants identified feeling more confident to have conversations about spirituality and pastoral care and being prepared to act differently themselves. However, the organization was reluctant to endorse this change and integrate spirituality and pastoral care. As one participant commented: '[In my area] there is a lack of understanding of how Pastoral Care can be integrated into the existing service, perhaps even a resistance.' Another said, 'this isn't seen as part of the role – more what pastors do, might be included in music therapy, volunteer role doing massage, not part of everybody's role'. Given this, these participants suggested it is hard to argue for time for ongoing education and reflection unless there is formal organizational change.

Beyond the dichotomy: learning from critical reflection individually and organizationally

Clearly, for some individuals in some organizations the learning from critical reflection does in itself generate change beyond the individual level, while others would say that the organization needs to more actively encourage this. Reynolds and Vince (2004, p. 1) support the need for a more organizational focus: 'reflection has been primarily concerned with individual rather than organization development ... Our view is that less emphasis needs to be placed on reflection as the task of individuals, and more emphasis needs to be on creating collective and organizationally focused processes for reflection'. This may mean organizations funding and endorsing the training and continued use of critical reflection processes and there are examples of this in Fook and Gardner (2013). Cressey, Boud and Docherty

(2006, p. 16) support a more organizational approach that initiates change rather than reflecting after the change has happened. What they call 'productive reflection' involves the 'creation of contextualized workplace learning that allows and releases the capacity of the workforce, via de-centralized and flexible project groups, the use of multi-functional networks and multiple stakeholder perspectives', with similarities to Wenger's (2000) communities of practice.

What is important here is not to create an unhelpful tension between individual reflection/change versus organizational reflection/change. Morley (2012) encourages moving beyond unhelpful dichotomies of seeing individual change versus system change and affirms that critical reflection reinforces that both are important. She used critical reflection processes as a research method to test the 'possibilities for change for practitioners engaged in supporting victims/survivors of sexual assault in the context of the Australian criminal justice system' (2012, p. 1513). She asked her research participants to bring a specific experience from their practice and as part of the research process worked with them through the two stages of critical reflection: deconstruction and reconstruction. What emerged was that the workers themselves found this process helpful in making links between their individual experience and feeling that it was possible to be more active about seeking some kind of systemic as well as individual change. Rose, for example, 'enhanced her capacity to exercise organization to create possibilities to challenge the legal system in ways that were rendered invisible by her initial discourses purely by a structural analysis' (Morley, 2012, p. 1530).

What does this suggest then? Fook (2010, p. 39) says:

> both realms (individual and organizational) are constructed by each other and of course both are influenced by the broader social context. What is important is to better understand this co-construction, in order to make organizational changes which are meaningful at both individual and organizational levels.

Change may be generated by individuals as well as from groups and formal structures, and it may be that organizations will be more responsive to structures that they have initiated –although there are no guarantees. Given that participants in critical reflection need to be emotionally engaged in the process, 'circumstances conducive to reflection need to be created' (Boud, 2010, p. 35). This also means having flexibility about opportunities for learning – and for critically reflecting, rather than a 'one-size-fits-all' mentality. Writing about 'situational leadership' and stages of movement from unconscious incompetence to conscious competence (Compton-Hall,

2003) reinforces that people change over time, so will have different preferences for learning.

The range of experiences articulated in Fook and Gardner (2013) reinforce the possibilities for change at an organizational and individual level by critically reflective processes adapted to the particular context. Sometimes organizations seek to bring about cultural change and will use critically reflective processes to do this. Critical reflection can also be used to 'research' practice in an organization, to identify what is working and what needs to change. Critically reflective processes can also be used as part of evaluation for specific projects in the organization or particular goals.

Using critical reflection to 'research practice' for change

What I mean by this is that a team or a group of people interested in the same issue can use a critically reflective process to articulate their knowledge about an aspect of their practice. This builds on Schön's (1983) view of the practitioner as researcher outlined in Chapter 1, evaluating and reflecting on experience to develop knowledge that might be called practice wisdom. The expectation is that all practitioners have knowledge about their practice, but it will be implicit and needs to be made explicit so that 'theories' or ideas about practice can be tested or further 'researched'. While individuals can of course do this on their own, it is often helpful to do this in a group where each person's contribution sparks contributions from others. The group can also provide a sense of what information is seen as shared or somewhat in common and what is more individual. There are several ways to do this and I outline three.

1. Using individual reflections to articulate group perspectives

One strategy is to work with a group or team with each individual initially presenting a significant experience that is then used to develop a group view. Critical reflection would be used in the usual way to enable this person to understand their experience at a deeper level. Once the individual has completed their reflection, you can then asked the group to articulate what has emerged from that person's reflection that says something about their own response, how does this person's experience connect to practice generally in the organization? As you work through the group, you start to build a rich picture of practice in this organization. It can help with this to focus the discussion on a particular area by asking each person to bring an experience that relates to a particular topic.

Thomson (2013) gives an example of this process in a community health organization where the critical reflection supervision group researched their community work practice. This group was made up of practitioners involved in community development and health promotion. One of their aims in having a critical reflection supervision group was to develop a shared theory of practice. Their hope was that if they became clearer about their practice as a group, they could more effectively share their approach to community work with the organization more broadly, and encourage the development of a community work approach across teams. The expectation was that their practice theory would also connect to formal community work and health promotion theory.

As the group worked through issues over time, they were able to articulate a shared theory of community development that was useful for constructively critiquing their own practice and wrestling with the challenges of offering community development and health promotion in an organization primarily focused on service provision. They presented their theory of practice to the whole staff group and to the organization's board of management and, as a result, were invited to provide training to other teams in the agency and to contribute this perspective to the organization's strategic plan.

Similarly, Gardner (2013) outlines the experience of participants in a mental health organization, where the effectiveness of supervision had been identified as an issue. The organization also wanted to implement supervision and critical reflection training for supervisors. Each participant was asked to bring an experience for their own reflection that related to supervision in the organization, wherever possible. Once each participant had completed their individual reflection, emerging issues, assumptions and values for the team and the organization were identified and listed on a white board. Of course, there was a range of experience, some very positive, some of frustration; some issues were more individually focused, but many related to organizational policies and processes or simply informal expectations that were unhelpful. They were written up so that they could be reviewed for the second stage of critical reflection and strategies for change identified.

The group used this to develop a series of principles for practice and then developed strategies, some of which required negotiation with the organizations. One issue was the lack of orientation for staff to new supervisors, particularly when a previous supervisor left either permanently or temporarily. When this was allied with such principles as: 'It is important to start supervision well – with expectations and ground rules, to have a process to fix things and to acknowledge what can and can't be fixed and where to go', it was clear that a strategy was needed to ensure appropriate orientation.

2. Focusing on a specific group issue: consumer consultation in mental health

Background: A particular community-based mental health team had been trying for several years to improve their inclusion of consumers in decision making about policy and practice in the organization and more broadly related to mental health services. The assumption was that it would be empowering for consumers to have the opportunity to participate. This had mainly taken the form of consultation about proposed changes, so meetings were held about specific issues that all consumers were invited to. However, the organization also had a consumer advisory group that met with the managers of the team on a regular basis.

Issue: Some of the consumers had expressed dissatisfaction about the consumer advisory group, feeling that their views were not effectively represented by the consumers that met with the managers and questioned how the consumers had been selected. The managers acknowledged that this had been quite an ad hoc process with team members asked to suggest interested consumers who would be confident to speak in meetings. This led to considerable angst in the team about effective consumer involvement and whether the espoused theory of empowering consumers was not theory in action. There were concerns that the current processes were tokenistic, and meant that consumers felt powerless, so either did not attend consultations or committee meetings or, if they did, did not feel able to contribute.

Process: The group of staff who were concerned about this issue met, bringing with them particular examples of their experience of trying to involve consumers in decision making for the organization. The key questions were: what works and what doesn't work? Most, but not all, of those in the group already had experience of using critical reflection in supervision. The aim was to work through a range of experiences, some positive others not, to identify common themes and develop these into principles for practice.

I will explore the first two experiences here and then the themes the group developed. We began with Helen's positive experience with a consumer called Jane who, two years previously, had asked to come to a consultation. Jane had been reluctant, feeling she wouldn't be able to say anything, but had agreed to attend the consultation on the basis that Helen would be there. Jane had, as she said, 'found her voice' and spoken so confidently that a manager had asked her to join the advisory group.

Initially, Helen found it very difficult to identify what might have made a difference, but said she knew Jane well before asking her to come to a consultation. As she talked more about this, she realized that often the pressure to find consumer representatives meant that she felt overly task focused in her relationships with consumers. Her assumption was that finding representatives was the priority. When she articulated this, and thought about the success of Jane's experience, she was able to suggest a new assumption that building relationships needs to come first. This led to her expressing a sense of unease about the limited ways in which consumers were able to express their views, which only suited a small number of consumers. This generated another assumption: consumer representatives need to fit with the current system of consultations and committees, rather than the system being flexible to fit consumer needs.

The next person to volunteer an experience in the group, Nick, had had a frustrating experience of inviting a consumer he thought was confident about speaking to the advisory group meeting. The consumer was both reluctant to speak and left halfway through the meeting. After hearing Helen's experience, he had realized that he had made several assumptions. First, that a consumer who was confident in giving their views with other consumers, would be equally confident in a formal meeting. Second, that no other training or support would be necessary for effective representation and third, that one consumer could reasonably be expected to speak on behalf of all other consumers. He said that hearing Helen's experience had been a 'light bulb' moment for him in that he could now see how unfair these assumptions were. He talked about his own challenges in getting his views across or even in feeling confident to speak in formal meetings where there were significant differences in power. He wondered why it was that he assumed that consumers with no training or support would feel more confident than someone like him who had considerable training and experience of organizational meetings.

This led in the group to the development of new assumptions or principles about how to more effectively include consumers in decision-making. These included:

- We need to build relationships with the consumers who are representatives so that there is a culture of mutual respect and support.
- To be effective representatives, consumers need training and support in meeting processes (access to these would mean greater sense of power).
- There needs to be a variety of ways in which consumers can participate in decision making in the organization.
- There needs to be more than one consumer in any meeting and preferably consumers should make up half of the group to shift the balance of power.
- To ensure a wider range of consumers can participate, we need funds for travel and childcare.

Each of the principles was then tested by the next experience and new assumptions/principles added or modified. As we went on, group members began to see patterns emerging and would briefly explain how their experience and assumptions connected. By the end of the session we had outlined a series of principles and the beginnings of a set of strategies that could be used to develop more effective forms of consultation. The group agreed to evaluate these in group interviews with consumers, then refine as needed.

3. Using critical reflection to research practice

This following framework was used with an organization called St Luke's in Victoria, Australia that wanted to encourage the development of a research culture. The research project aimed at identifying factors that would support the development of the organization's capacity to carry out research and enhance a 'culture of inquiry' (Gardner and Nunan, 2007). Two teams volunteered to take part in a collaborative critically reflective research approach using the following questions to guide discussion and implementation of the research. This set of questions can also be used as a framework to explore a particular issue. Instead of using specific experiences as you would do in a critical reflection supervision group, the questions have embedded in them assumptions from the critical reflection process – such as the importance of exploring different views on a particular issue. The questions also connect to the stages of a more traditionally named research project: 'The development of the research question, a literature review and methodology'.

Critically reflective questions for researching practice

What is the issue to be explored? How is it constructed as a problem?
- Who sees it as a problem?
- What variety of views is there?
- What specifically do people want to consider?
- What are the underlying assumptions and values?
- Why now? Why has it come up as an issue now?
- What is the history of this issue?
- What policy/context aspects are there?
- Are there a range of views about the background? What impact does that have on how the issue is now being seen?

Has the issue been thought about by other people?
- What did they think?
- What conclusions did they come to?
- What questions did they raise?

Why are workers interested in this issue?
- o What range of views is there?
- o What do workers hope will happen?
- o What do workers know from their experience?
- o What do workers assume from their experience?

What needs to be asked/explored? What kind of information is needed? For example, specific or general questions and prompts, factual information vs views/ideals/beliefs?
- o What voices need to be heard about the issue?
- o Are there particular voices likely to be harder to access?
- o How will you make sure these are heard?

How will people be involved?
- o What ways of asking people for information are likely to work with these groups, particularly people experiencing the issue?
- o What resources are available? What timelines are there?
- o What ethical issues might there be and how can they be managed?

Two groups of staff volunteered to use this approach. One group, the Youth Team, wanted to provide services for young sexual offenders. Initially, the team experienced some frustration with the research process and the critically reflective questions as they opened up the complexities of the potential research question. The team had seen the research as focusing on how to provide specific services for this service-user group given their collective experience of resource gaps. In practice, exploring the question meant asking: 'Whose problem is this?', 'How differently is it perceived by different communities of interest?', 'Is the issue about the community's reaction rather than the need for more services?'. This was initially perceived as delaying what was needed. Having a student to carry out a literature review helped generate a sense of achievement and understanding of the variety of views and evidence. It was decided to begin by having a day with other service providers to gather perspectives on the issue.

The overall evaluation of the project (creating a culture of inquiry in the organization) found that those interviewed from across the organization thought there was a sense of cultural change in their teams and the organization generally: first greater reflection about practice: 'more stopping to "think, question, ask what happens and why?"' (Gardner and Nunan, 2007, p. 342). In both project teams, reflection became part of the agenda of team meetings 'as a strategy to explore and address issues, such as thinking about policy development'. If an issue arose, participants were more likely to want to think through the issues rather than simply reacting. Some felt that this cultural change would be empowering for staff and service users, generating more effective practices:

'a change from seeing evaluation/research as extra work to seeing it as helping reflection and in the long term meaning more time with service users'.

This project was helped by the organization allocating funds for a research project worker who was able to actively support the teams. It does demonstrate that change is possible in an organization's culture using critically reflective processes supported by the organization and where staff can volunteer to participate in teams – or contextualized work groups.

Evaluating your practice as a worker

Being critically reflective is in itself a way of building in evaluation: a form of constantly checking your assumptions and values, the possibilities of thinking/acting/reacting in different ways. It can be helpful though to more formally build this into practice, partly to check that you and your practice are being perceived in the ways you think you are.

Much evaluation is of the kind where people tick boxes about levels of satisfaction. This clearly only gives limited information and often doesn't address the more complex issues of what has been helpful. As a practitioner, it is useful to think about developing your own form of evaluation, asking what it is that you want to understand from those that you are working with and how you might ask in a way that means you are more likely to get that information. This might mean building in evaluation questions at the end of a session or a number of sessions that become part of how you work together. You might ask, for example, what is it that is helpful in this process? Asking such a question, from a position of genuine interest, helps both you and the service user or community reach a deeper understanding about what aspects of your work together are effective from their perspective.

Examples of possible questions:

o What were you expecting/ hoping for?
o What was helpful about what did happen? (what did you learn that you would use?)
o What would you have liked to be different?
o What would you say to someone else interested in coming to ...?

Summary

This chapter engaged with the issue of how critical reflection can be used to influence organizations and their practices. Individual reflection and action can bring about change, but organizational commitment makes a significant difference to embedding critical reflection and emerging learning. Several strategies for using critical reflection to generate organizational change have been explored: combining the learning from individual reflections in groups; focusing on using critical reflection experiences related to a particular issue; and research and evaluation practice using critical reflection understanding.

Questions for reflection

- Think about a time when you experienced change in an organization.
- What was your reaction? What was it influenced by?
- What did or could have helped you to see this experience of change as an opportunity for learning?
- What are your preferred strategies for change? Why? What has this been influenced by?
- How might you use critically reflective processes to generate change – for yourself and for the organization? How might these overlap?

6 Supervision and Team Work

It can be hard to be critically reflective on your own. Assumptions and values can be so deeply embedded that it is challenging to unearth them, to ask yourself the kinds of questions that elicit feelings and thoughts that are uncomfortable. This chapter explores the use of supervision in developing and maintaining a critically reflective stance to practice. First, ideas about supervision in general are explored, including the development of common themes about supervision across disciplines. Traditional ways of thinking about supervision are identified: the combination of accountability, support and educational roles in a one-to-one relationship between a more senior staff member and a more junior one. Instead thinking about supervision as how professional practice is effectively supported can lead to more flexible and creative arrangements: asking how supervision needs can be negotiated to suit the individual and the organization. The aim here is to encourage practitioners to think more broadly about their own assumptions about how they are supervised and how they are supported to be critically reflective in their organization and what their preferences might be. The differences between individual, group and peer supervision are explored as well as the benefits of these for individual practitioners and for changing organizational culture towards being more critically reflective. This leads to exploring the potential to think of supervision as a way of embedding critical reflection in organizational and in practice through using critical reflection in individual and group supervision, for example.

Different perceptions of supervision

Professionals attending critical reflection workshops have mixed reactions to supervision, usually from their experience of it and this is reflected in the varied perceptions of supervision in the literature. Some see supervision as a constructive and supportive way to explore practice and professional issues. For others, the word itself has negative connotations related to power differences: of being scrutinized or overseen, as one participant said: 'super-vision – yuk!', explaining that he preferred a more collegial, egalitarian style.

A more managerialist approach combined with changes in the labour market has led to such questions as whether a professional needs to be supervised by someone from the same discipline. There are also questions about whether there is sufficient inclusion of differences in personality and learning style and so the need to match supervisor and supervisee. Learning and professional development is now seen as lifelong and writers suggest the value of including more experiential and reflective practices. There are issues too about providing supervision across disciplines, when supervision should be discipline specific and when interdisciplinary supervision is advantageous. Finally, traditional supervision practices may not sufficiently acknowledge the influence of both organizational and social context on both the processes and content discussed in supervision.

Supervision has also been perceived quite differently depending on the discipline with some professions having supervision systems firmly established and others only recently considering how supervision might be included in practice. Traditionally, supervision has been more embedded in some professions than others such as social work (Kadushin,1985; Brown and Bourne, 1995), psychology (Fleming and Steen, 2011), psychotherapy (Bager-Charleson, 2010) and nursing (Bishop, 1998; Driscoll, 2000), but is increasingly seen as part of professional practice for other disciplines such as occupational therapy (Gaitskell and Morley, 2008), speech therapy (Geller, 2001) or allied health generally (Rose and Best, 2005). This is reflected in the increase of writing on supervision across disciplines rather than for a particular discipline, such as Hawkins and Shohet (2006) writing for the 'helping professions' or Rolfe, Jasper and Freshwater (2011) for 'generating knowledge for care'. This increased interest is partly a response to greater interest in quality and risk management. Research also suggests that aspects of supervision such as task assistance, social and emotional support and positive interpersonal interactions are related to beneficial outcomes for workers and so also to organizations in terms of retention and quality of work (Barak et al., 2009). More specifically rapport between supervisor and supervisee links strongly with job satisfaction across disciplines (Mena and Bailey, 2007).

While greater interest in supervision is reflected in the literature, how it is defined and the language used is not always consistent. Bond and Holland's definition (1998, p. 12) makes clear that the primary aim of supervision is high-quality practice. It focuses on the traditional perception of supervision between a worker who is less experienced and a more experienced colleague probably at a more senior level in the organization:

Clinical supervision is regular, protected time for facilitated, in depth reflection on clinical practice. It aims to enable the supervisee to achieve, sustain and creatively develop a high quality of practice through the means of focused support and development. The supervisee reflects on the part she plays as an individual in the complexities of the events and quality of her practice. This reflection is facilitated by one or more experienced colleagues who have expertise in facilitation.

Hawkins and Shohet (2006, p. 5) suggest that supervision 'is an indispensable part of the helper's wellbeing, ongoing self-development, self-awareness and commitment to development' and also that supervision 'is not a straightforward process and is even more complex than working with service users'. Seeing the supervisory process as collaborative is part of Wood and Schuck's definition (2011, p. 12) focusing on

> the personal and professional development of one of them. The supervisory process is in itself a creative process because it involves a deep and multi-faceted reflective engagement by the supervisee that is triggered by apt and timely questioning by the supervisor

or in groups by comments and questions from other group members.

Some organizations focus on 'clinical' supervision or specific issues related to a professional discipline as opposed to organizational or management supervision; in other organizations staff have access to or are expected to have both kinds of supervision. Some staff find this valuable (Gardner, 2013) and suggest that having a supervisor from a different discipline opens up other perspectives and this is supported by the literature (Fronek et al., 2009).

However, this may partly relate to who the supervisor is. Chipchase et al. (2012) found, admittedly with a small group of students also working across cultures, that students found it helpful to have both discipline specific and interdisciplinary supervision. Oelofsen, a psychologist (2012, p. 176) equates 'clinical' and 'case' supervision, which he conceptualizes 'as a set of spaces which provides the time and place for practitioners to reflect … as a narrative space (where the stories of services, practitioners, and service users intersect), supervision as a space to think, and supervision as a space for enactment and containment'. This language also suggests the potential to use different theoretical approaches as part of supervision, from the narrative to the psychodynamic. What is meant by clinical varies and an issue with the clinical definition of supervision can be its lack of attention to the 'critical' or inclusion of social context, which is, of course, included in critically reflective supervision.

What is agreed about supervision

Three key functions

What is agreed about supervision is first that it is of value and second that there are three key aspects or functions of supervision (Kadushin, 1985; Proctor, 2008). The language used for these varies but they are essentially:

- *Management/accountability/qualitative*: this is often seen as the quality control aspect of supervision that ensures a high quality of practice in line with organizational goals. It includes the practical nuts and bolts of supervision such as reviewing existing work, allocating new work, discussions about leave and other organizational requirements.
- *Supportive/restorative/resourcing*: this is the enabling, encouraging, regenerating side of supervision. This particularly requires a relationship of trust so that it is possible to reflect more deeply on practice, to explore emotions, doubts, possibilities, to debrief. In this aspect of supervision, personal, professional, organizational and contextual issues can be explored, including the dynamic in supervision itself. This may also include broad questions like: How are you going overall? How are you feeling about work? How are you managing busyness/stress?
- *Educational/formative/developmental*: there is also a teaching and learning aspect of supervision, provision of relevant knowledge, learning and/or practising new skills through demonstration or explanation.

Centrality of reflective practices

What is also agreed about supervision is that reflective practice or critical reflection is crucial. Freshwater (2011b, p. 103) sees supervision and reflective practice as interdependent: 'clinical supervision can be described as a flexible and dynamic structure within which to continuously deconstruct and reconstruct clinical practice. Fundamental to this process of deconstruction and reconstruction are the skills of reflection, critical reflection and reflexivity'. Noble and Irwin (2009, p. 354) argue that the 'critical' aspect of critical reflection will encourage 'supervision sessions [to] address the impact of power differentials associated with gender, class and ethnicity, as well as cultural and other structural barriers and their impact on the function and process of supervision'. Thinking critically helps make explicit practitioners and the organization's underlying assumptions and how these influence actions. 'A critical lens will explore and reflect on the way the supervisors, the supervisees and the organizations work with the service users/service users and this reflection will help practitioners make their actions and those of the organization more explicit and conscious.' Patel (2011, p. 102) suggests that supervision is one of the main sites in organizations where power and related differences are experienced and need to be addressed. Her concern is focused on differences in ethnic background between supervisor and supervisee where 'the majority ethnic supervisor's anxieties about their competence in understanding and addressing issues of power, culture, ethnicity and racism may be compounded by the minority supervisee's anxieties about how they will be negatively evaluated or misunderstood by the supervisor because of their minority ethnic status'. She suggests that statements like 'I treat everyone the same', are inherently unhelpful, demonstrating a lack of understanding of what it means to be in a minority. Her comments can apply to many other aspects of 'difference' and affirm the need for critically reflective awareness.

Supervision and critical reflection: making active choices

What is helpful in sustaining a critically reflective attitude to practice, is to move from a more traditional understanding of supervision or from acceptance of what an organization offers to asking: How can I best ensure that my supervision needs are met? How can I make sure that I am an effective practitioner? Rather than necessarily expecting one supervisor to combine the three aspects of supervision: management; supportive/restorative and educational/developmental, asking what combination of support or encouragement, challenge or training will best suit me? There are no 'right' answers to what kind of supervision will work best. Clearly the answers to these questions will vary over time depending on your level of experience, personality, skills and confidence as well as what options and choices there are in your organization or in the broader context.

This can necessitate a change in thinking both individually and organizationally. Noble and Irwin (2009, p. 356) suggest that in the current economic landscape:

> taken for granted assumptions, approaches and methods currently informing supervision need revisiting in order to open up creative spaces in the way supervision is practiced and can be practiced. The time is right to take on this challenge and open up supervision to a more critically reflective analysis in order to allow space for new strategies and responses to emerge.

Traditionally, for example, one supervisor, who was usually also the line manager, took on all three of these roles and this continues to be the case in some organizations. There are some advantages in this if it is working well. Having one manager means that the three functions are easily integrated. Supposing, for example, I am working in palliative care and am supervising someone who tells me from a supportive/restorative perspective that she is feeling very stressed by her mother's life threatening illness, combined with an adolescent doing final exams. I can then easily, from my management perspective, decide to postpone suggesting changes in work practice or taking on new work and from an educational perspective suggest a stress management course. On the other hand, because of the complexities of power, some practitioners will not feel safe to disclose feeling personally and/or professionally challenged to a supervisor who will also be assessing their performance for pay increments or promotion. Others may feel that their line manager does not have the particular skills or knowledge that they would prefer for support or for their professional development. For these reasons, some organizations already separate these roles: one individual might have a line manager, that is, the person above them in the hierarchy for 'accountability' supervision, a discipline or clinical supervisor for supportive/restorative supervision and the education aspect might be arranged through a separate training unit. The disadvantage of this can be that the supervisee needs to decide whether to repeat information to different supervisors so that their issues are understood. Alternatively, the supervisor/s and supervisee need to clarify under what circumstances each will share information with the other.

Supervision as a team or group

The traditional one-to-one model of supervision is also being challenged by the development of group supervision. Group supervision of some kind can be very effective for team development creating what Ghaye (2005) calls teams as 'communities of learners' and Wenger (2000) 'communities of practice' as discussed in the previous chapter. There are various forms of group supervision: peer supervision is where colleagues at the same level meet usually for supportive/restorative and/or educational/developmental supervision. The group may meet for case discussion combined with mutual support or, of course, use something like the two-stage critical reflection process. Peer supervision removes some of the aspects of power that can be unhelpfully present in other forms of supervision, no one is making decisions about anyone else's management. However, of course, other forms of power may be present – such as the influence of personality, length of experience in the workplace or perceived influence. Occasionally I have experienced having a manager join a peer supervision groups, with mixed success. Thinking about reflexivity is useful here: some managers and their supervisees are able to suspend their role perceptions of each other to be equal participants in peer group supervision, and when this is successful it can mean a greater sense of shared power outside the group. On the other hand, the manger's role can get in the way. A group member may wonder whether a manger will continue to be influenced outside the group by their sharing of their feelings of inadequacy about a particular experience. This then inevitably affects the openness of the discussion. Baker (2013) explores the complexities of this in a statutory setting where the institutionalized power imbalances between himself as manager and workers in the group made critical reflection particularly challenging.

Group supervision is more likely to include a manager particularly if it is for team supervision rather than peer supervision. Group supervision might include information sharing, case or issue discussion, mutual support and/or critical reflection. Including critical reflection where individuals are expected to share specific examples may be complicated by including a manger as described above, but it may be that critically reflective processes can be used in the team in other ways – such as discussing shared issues or 'researching practice' as described in the previous chapter. With either kind of group it is essential to clarify and seek agreement about the aims of the group, how it will be run and what the decision-making processes will be.

There are many benefits as well as challenges of group critical reflection for supervision and these have been explored in a range of organizations in Fook and Gardner (2013) including in voluntary (Thomson, 2013) and statutory settings (Ferguson, 2013) and in student supervision (Allan, 2013). Given that critical reflection is asking participants to share challenging aspects of their work and they may well feel vulnerable, it is important that all group members feel able to trust each other, including that material discussed in the group will not be used in any kind of negative way outside the group. The supervision group described by Thomson (2013) is particularly concerned about this issue and identifies early in the process their expectation that anything discussed in the group will not be mentioned by anybody outside the group, unless the person whose experience it is chooses to do so. If critical reflection is part of the group process, an appropriate culture needs to be established (as discussed in Chapter 1). It also helps to have a facilitator for the group, either an external facilitator skilled in critical reflection if funding allows or to have group members take on the role. The facilitator's role is to concentrate on making sure the culture of critical reflection is working well, asking the group to stop and reflect on the culture and process if necessary.

Critical reflection in group supervision can enhance teamwork, group members feeling that they understand and value to a greater degree what other group members bring to a team. Ferguson (2013, p. 91) found that simply feeling listened to was helpful, but more specifically 'workers reflecting that they feel more self-aware, and have developed a greater understanding of colleagues which has led to a more meaningful understanding of their team and how it can function'. Peer supervision using critical reflection can work across disciplines providing a common language for people to share experiences (Gardner and Taalman, 2013). Welsh and Dehler (2004, p. 15) suggest that groups, such as critical reflection supervision groups, 'hold greater potential to transform organizations by institutionalizing democratic practices'. Certainly the experience of critical reflection groups over time demonstrates first that they generate acceptance and mutual respect and decision making and can also influence constructively seeking organizational change (Thomson, 2013).

Being creative about supervision

Once you start thinking about how supervision needs will be met rather than only using existing structures, other possibilities abound, both formal and informal, funded and unfunded. Some participants from critical reflection workshops have chosen to meet for mutual support/restoration with a colleague once a month for an hour. Each person takes it in turns to present an experience and explore it for half an hour. In another group, participants agreed that colleagues could request a 'critical reflection' lunch or coffee when they wanted some supervision about a particular experience. Some people choose to seek external supervision: someone outside their organizations with particular skills and/or knowledge. Occasionally an organization will fund this particularly if there is a view that no one in the organization has these skills, but some participants fund this themselves. If organizations are funding external supervision they are likely to want some kind of agreement about reporting back particularly if there are concerns about professional standards. Informal supervision is also another, often unrecognized, way of meeting supervision needs: casual conversations possibly in the tea room or in passageways or across desks that provide information, opportunities for debriefing or quick reflection. Some people use journaling (see Chapter 3) and use their findings or remaining questions in individual or peer supervision. Others are developing forms of mutual supervision, in the sense used here, using blogs, Skyping or a range of other digital practices. These can have the advantage of being outside the organization so more egalitarian and some of these can be anonymous.

Organizations may also offer opportunities that can be part of a desired supervision 'package', especially for developmental/educational needs. Larger organizations often have a calendar of training activities. Most expect that professionals need to maintain their knowledge and skills through continuing education and professional development. Being critically reflective can heighten awareness of what you want or need and the confidence to find out what education and training is available and ask for it. Some organizations build in opportunities for learning through seminars, case discussions across disciplines, speakers on relevant topics, some of which can happen without extra funding. Organizations do vary in how much they fund education/development activities, and this will also vary depending on the funding context. The challenge in a restricted funding environment can be to find ways around this, to look for possibilities for mutual sharing of knowledge and skills across organizations. It might be that a training session with an outside facilitator could be funded by opening up training to other organizations, for example.

Also now recognized is the need for the supervisor and supervisee to understand and seek to work with their differences in personality, learning style, experience, skills levels and relevant aspects of their personal and professional history, differences in beliefs and values and the assumptions that have developed from these, that is, the need to be critically reflective, of their own assumptions and those in the organization. Organizational cultures vary in how much this is accepted, for example, whether the norm is 'people have to accept and manage to work with the allocated supervisor' or 'people can have some choice about who their supervisor is'.

How can each person ensure their particular supervision needs are met?

The question then becomes how can you generate your own preferred supervision combination – and of course this will need to change over time.
It helps to ask yourself questions like:

- What is it that I find helpful/appropriately challenging for this stage of my working life?
- How do I want to be supported, questioned, enabled, regenerated?
- What are the assumptions I make in relation to supervision?
  - About myself?
  - About others?
- How have I been influenced by past experience?
  - Of my own?
  - Of others?
- What is the variety of ways rather than one way?
- How am I being influenced by the organizational context?
  - What does or can this organization offer?
  - What assumptions am I making about these?

- What other options do I have?
- How can I access these? What do I need to do now to act on this?

It may be useful to discuss these with another person – in the spirit of critical friendship to help draw out what is assumed and what might be possible.

Examples of using critical reflection in supervision

Clearly being critically reflective can be an attitude to supervision that permeates any form of supervision or mutually supportive relationships. Alternatively, the two-stage critical reflection process or other processes outlined in Chapter 3 can be used. Whatever processes are used, it is important that all those involved are clear about the process and how it works and that the culture of critical reflection is established with a sense of trust and acceptance.

The following three cases studies highlight particular aspects of using critical reflection explicitly in supervision: the first relates to using critical reflection to deconstruct what supervision itself means for a particular person. Reflecting critically about supervision itself can elicit assumptions about how supervision or supervisors/supervisees 'should be'. Deconstructing these assumptions can open up new possibilities. Here I have used Claire's example to explore her perception of supervision and supervisors and how these changed as she used critical reflection. The second example is of a supervisor and supervisee using critical reflection to understand more fully a particular experience from a community development perspective. The third example considers reactions in a peer group supervision and the particular difficulty of managing the reactions of others in the group when they are different from the person with the experience.

Claire's experience

Background: I am the supervisor of a small nursing team in a large health service. We were having trouble managing a waiting list and I had what I thought was a great idea how to manage this. I had already had several discussions with my supervisor, Peta but we hadn't come up with anything the organization would agree to.

The experience: I called in to see Peta and mentioned my idea; to my surprise and outrage really, she just dismissed the idea.

Why it was significant: I felt really let down that my idea hadn't even been properly listened to, I thought I'd come up

Case study 6.1

with something that was worthwhile and should have been given more time.

Stage one

As Claire teased out her reactions what emerged was that she felt undermined. Her experience felt symbolic of how Peta treated her. After more exploration, which seemed to be getting stuck on Claire's frustration with Peta, she was asked what assumptions she had about supervisors. Claire responded supervisors should always listen, be patient, be open, supportive, encouraging to their supervisees, give constructive criticism where necessary, but always balance this with positive feedback. She thought this was her assumption about how she should act as a supervisor too. One of the group members said 'so the supervisor has to be perfect then?' Claire laughed but then agreed and said it was a difficult image to live up to. She found it hard to perceive Peta in any way but a source of frustration, but agreed it would be useful to idea storm where Peta might be coming from. The group generated a list of possibilities:

- Peta has no supervision experience and hates being a supervisor.
- Peta is under pressure to succeed in the role so is stressed about suggesting anything seen as unworkable.
- Peta prefers working on her own, but is using this job as a stepping stone to something else.
- Peta is stressed by something in her personal life and it's coming out at work.

While Claire didn't know if any of these were accurate, they shifted her perception of her supervisor and supervision. She acknowledged that she had expected Peta to be superhuman and that by implication she expected the same of herself. She began to explore possible new assumptions:

- Supervisors are human too.
- They have good and bad days.
- They will be influenced by what else is happening for them.
- Supervisors vary; have different levels of experience and skills.
- Supervisors aren't always able to respond well on the spot.

- Supervisors will be influenced by what else is happening in the organization.

Stage two

When Claire returned for stage two, she told the group that she had felt somehow freed by the discussion and raised her concern with Peta, saying she had felt undermined by her reaction and that even if the idea had no merit, she would like to feel respected for trying to come up with a solution. Peta had apologized, saying that she felt she was feeling very stressed by the expectations of the job combined with caring for small children. This experience clarified for Claire that she had made another assumption: that she was powerless in relation to supervision and her relationship with Peta. She now felt she had acted in an empowered way: her new assumption was that she could act to bring about change.

From exploring organizational expectations of supervisors, Claire realized that she had internalized cultural and organizational norms reinforced by her own high standards of work practice. The 'expectation of perfection' was wearing for her too. She decided she needed to develop new assumptions particularly 'supervisors are human too' and 'supervisors also have needs'. Recognizing that not all her supervision needs would be met by Peta, she decided to seek mentoring from a manager in another section and to explore whether peer critical reflection could be developed. Finally, she decided to use a phrase that had come up several times in discussion: 'what is reasonable' to remind herself to be open to possibilities without expecting perfection.

Pat's experience

Background: I was working as a community worker in a rural neighbourhood house, established to encourage the then current government's community capacity building initiative, a base to develop skills and activities in the local community, including some adult education and access to computers. One of the issues the

Case study 6.2

community group managing the house had wanted to address was the lack of children's play equipment in the park next door. Over a couple of years, I had supported the group to develop skills in negotiating with the local council. They had been successful in receiving funding and a play area with brightly coloured creative structures, combined with swings and slides had been created primarily aimed at young children.

Experience: I was the last to leave the house one early evening and noticed that a group of young adolescent boys were playing on the structure and that one had a can of spray and had started to graffiti the slide. I felt really angry and ran over to them shouting at them to stop what they were doing or I would call the police. Most of them ran away, but the one with the spray threatened to spray me, I took my phone out of my bag, he went to snatch it, but at that moment there was a shout from a passing community group member and he ran off.

Significant: I was horrified at how angry my reaction was, it was really over the top and especially what I had shouted at them and what I thought about them.

Stage one

Pat clarified that she didn't have any question that what the boys were doing was wrong and needed to stop. What she felt uncomfortable about was how quickly she identified with the judgemental attitudes of many in the local community. The community group had suggested having parents/committee members to patrol the area and make sure it wasn't vandalized and she had felt that was an over-reaction, based on critical assessments of people in the community. In the heat of the moment, and the immediate aftermath, she found herself making the same assessments: these people are a waste of space, what's the point of doing anything in a community where people are so hopeless, these kids should be locked up or taught a lesson of some kind. What happened, she asked to her values of respect, valuing all individuals, understanding the influence of background and social context, how could she slip so quickly into negativity. How had her espoused values so dramatically not been expressed in action? Why hadn't she approached them as a community worker and at least tried to talk to them?

In exploring this further, Pat recognized that some of her anger was on behalf of the local group who had worked hard for this and with whom she worked. She identified more with them than she had realized. She also felt a contradictory combination of reactions. First maybe the committee was right and I was wrong, we should have patrolled the park and reflexively, the committee will certainly now perceive me as wrong and that implies my values are wrong. At the same time, she wanted to assert other values from a critical, postmodern perspective – I do understand that those young boys may feel resentful, they are marginalized, their voice the least heard. She also felt somewhat shaken by the potential for violence, but as she explored this, more by the anger, maybe hatred in the boy's expression. Taking reflexively further, she could see that from his perspective, she was one of the community that see him as hopeless, and to her shame, in that moment, she was. She asked 'why would they assume I'd be any different with them from others in the group?'

Stage two

This took Pat to articulating and affirming her assumptions: everyone is of value and has their reasons for their reactions – which applied to her as well as others. She realized she had become somewhat seduced by the group's dichotomies of community members into being 'good and bad' and that she needed to stand back from this and continue to espouse a different perspective. Connected to this was seeing that most of her energy had been influenced by the committee to focus on younger children and families and older people. She decided the voice of older children and adolescents, about their perceptions and preferences for community change, needed to be heard while acknowledging that she couldn't assume they would see her as approachable. She decided she wanted to affirm her assumptions and values and act from them.

There are many examples of using group supervision in the critical reflection literature (Fook and Gardner, 2013). Although the detail of how the group operates will vary, essentially, a group of about 6–8 meet about monthly for two hours. Group members take it in turn to present an experience that has been significant to them in some way: perhaps bothered, intrigued, annoyed, puzzled. Depending on the group and the time available, usually one or two people will present, but may only present one stage in the session and complete the second stage at the next session or may complete both stages in an hour and move on to the second person. The group generally has a facilitator; some groups would also have a timekeeper and/or a note taker. The note taker might write on a whiteboard key comments/issues and this is often helpful for externalizing what has been said and with remembering it. These roles rotate in the group and groups develop their own expectations about when the changes happen. Some groups like to organize a schedule of who will present for six months or a year ahead; others decide at the end of each session. What does seem to be important in maintaining momentum is planning dates ahead and sticking to them. The process is described in more detail in Fook and Gardner (2007).

I have chosen to use an example here that illustrates a particular aspect of how this works: what might be called synchronicity in a team. Often when one person describes their experience, it will resonate with others in the team, which can then provide useful learning for others. Part of the learning in the group is understanding that people may react differently to the same experience or that people may have similar reactions but from different assumptions. What can also happen of course is that people react strongly to a similar experience with the danger then being that they find it hard not to impose their perspective on others. Working with this as a whole group can increase learning overall about how to use critical reflection to build the team's understanding of professional practice.

David's experience

Case study 6.3

Background: I had been working as a supervisor for about 18 months including supervising a relatively new graduate Donna.

Experience: Donna told me that our manager had asked her if she would prefer to be supervised by someone else. She told the manager, Ken, that she was happy with my supervision. We talked it over and I felt confident that Donna was happy with my supervision, but I now feel uncomfortable about why Ken asked Donna about changing.

Significance: This has left me feeling uneasy with Ken, I still wonder why he asked, but because Donna gave him her answer, I feel I shouldn't question him, that that would undermine Donna being seen as being able to do this for herself.

Stage one

When asked to say more about how he felt David identified again his discomfort with Ken's action. Because the group resonated strongly with this, discussion stuck on the reasonableness of his response. Eventually, someone asked what the assumption was here: this elicited David's assumption that Ken was being critical of his supervision. Once he had articulated that he laughed and said he was surprised that was his first assumption and wondered why he had been so 'paranoid'. He connected this with rumours of a restructure and possible redundancies. Asked how he would generally respond to conflict, he acknowledged that he preferred to avoid conflict. He suggested though that this was not the central issue for him, it was that he had so quickly assumed that there must be something wrong with his supervision.

At this point, two of the other group members: Rose and Grace asked such questions as 'but don't you think you need to challenge the manager yourself?', 'Isn't it now important to find out what is happening here?' When the facilitator for the session (another group member) reminded them about the culture of respect, they could see that they were reacting from their own assumptions and past experiences rather than hearing David's and that their questions implied negative judgement of David.

Stage two

David reiterated that he wanted to explore more the assumptions he had made and how to shift them. He thought his assumption initially was: 'this must be to do with me; it must be my fault'. This connected for him to the uncertainty in the organization and to his past experience of redundancy. At a conscious level, he understood that this was not personal, he had been the last person employed, and others, more senior, had been made redundant too as a result of government cuts. When asked so what then influenced this feeling, he eventually realized that he had internalized negative messages about being unemployed from his father particularly, but also friends, general comments in shops and in the media. In retrospect, he felt this influenced him to be less assertive than usual and more likely to blame himself. The group worked with him to generate new assumptions such as 'this is not about me' and possible strategies such as asking 'so what is really happening here?' These he planned to use as his 'slogans' to prompt him to come from a different perspective if something similar happened and to ask directly and constructively about what was happening.

Group discussion: Once Dave felt he was finished, the group decided to explore the process in general, particularly Rose and Grace's reaction. Rose and Grace related examples of feeling abused by a past supervisor. Neither had received any support from their more senior managers in spite of raising these issues several times. The culture of the organization was 'don't rock the boat' or 'it's too hard to change things like this' and they had to some degree internalized this culture. One had eventually left the organization, the other outlasted her supervisor. Because of these experiences they now felt much more strongly that something should be done and this was the basis of their reaction to David.

When the group talked about these experiences collectively, the discussion moved between exploring the organization's dominant culture and the assumptions of individuals and how these were influenced by the social context in a broader way. For Rose and Grace this felt partly gender related – the 'don't be a woman making a fuss about nothing' they experienced socially. This left them in a state of tension because they felt disempowered and that this was inconsistent with their values and what organizational values should be. The group articulated some collective assumptions that were affirming for both of these workers, that everyone agreed might lead to more mutual support if this situation happened again:

- that abusive behaviour is unacceptable,
- organizations have a responsibility for the safety of their workers, and
- I am justified in taking action to ensure that I am in a supportive and helpful workplace.

They also affirmed the importance of each group member being conscious of their reactions to someone else's experience and to at least temporarily, set these aside to let the person with the experience explore their perspective.

Summary

This chapter explored how supervision can be used to support being critically reflective. A broader way of thinking about supervision is to ask: What are my supervision needs: my needs for support, challenge, learning? How can these enable critically reflective processes to become part of my working life? Thinking flexibly about supervision allows for the range of possibilities explored in the chapter: individual supervision, peer and group supervision, informal and formal, internal and external complemented by specific training as needed.

Questions for reflection

- What experiences of supervision have you had? What was your reaction to these – what were your thoughts, feelings, the development of related assumptions? What was it about these experiences that worked? What would you want to change?
- How would you describe your current preferences/needs for supervision in the sense of management, support/enabling and educational/training?
- What sorts of creative strategies could you use/develop to meet these?
- How could you build critically reflective processes into the kind/s of supervision that you prefer?

Critical Reflection and the Broader Professional Context

7 Ethical Issues

The ethics of practice are confronting for all professional disciplines in their practice as well as in general organizational life (Banks, 2008; Jensen, Royeen and Purtilo, 2010; Laabs, 2011). These dilemmas are often expressed by practitioners as stresses or conflict, sometimes conflict with service users, but more often with colleagues or managers. This may relate to simply having a colleague that is experienced as being difficult to work with or a specific disagreement or dispute that is named as an ethical or moral difference. The possible scope of these is endless and to some extent what is ethically challenging is subjective: some people will experience a particular issue as an ethical dilemma that others see as straightforward. For some workers, the resulting stress leads to ongoing discomfort or for some, burnout and leaving the organization and/or the profession. Critical reflection can provide a process for identifying ethical issues and unearthing assumptions and values that may contribute to feeling 'stuck' with them, accessing other ways of seeing what is happening and finding ways to either resolve, manage or live with the conflict.

The inevitability of engaging with ethical dilemmas is certainly reinforced in critical reflection workshops. Practitioners often connect being ethical with maintaining a sense of integrity about how they approach practice. Banks (2010, p. 2171) outlines three versions of what she calls professional integrity developed from interviews with senior practitioners in the social welfare field. These are first: morally good or right conduct, focusing on doing what is professionally right; as commitment to a set of deeply held values. Second, Banks suggests standing up for what is believed to be right, and third: the capacity to be continuously reflexive in seeking to evaluate and make sense of actions. She suggests (p. 2180) that no one of these is enough on its own, what is needed is 'critical awareness of how the concept of professional integrity is being used' as well as the capacity to be reflexive both in seeking to understand 'moral motivations and commitments of professional practitioners' and their relationship to their work. A possible framework for this includes focusing on values and beliefs: being able to name professional and personal values and how these interrelate, and to be able to explain these to others. Banks (2008, p. 1244) also makes explicit that ethical issues 'cannot be abstracted from the political and policy context in which they take place.'

Codes of practice and their application

Professional disciplines do all, of course, have codes of ethics or expectations of professional practice and these reflect the discipline's values. Owens, Springwood and Wilson 2012, p. 30) summarize what they see as principles across professional organizations: 'non-maleficence (do no harm), benefi-cence (increasing well-being), justice, autonomy, fidelity, respect and self-respect. Clark in Pierson (2002, p. 21) summarizes four broad principles related to social work ethics: '1. The worth and uniqueness of every person ... 2. Entitlement to justice ... 3. Claim to freedom: every person and social group is entitled to their own beliefs and pursuits unless it restricts the free-dom of others. 4. Community is essential to human life.' Other disciplines have much in common with these, with some being more specific than others: the Canadian Nurses Association Code (2008) includes providing safe, compassionate, competent care; promoting health and wellbeing; promoting and respecting informed decision making; preserving dignity; maintaining privacy and confidentiality; promoting justice and being accountable. Codes of ethics provide practitioners with a clear and often inspirational value base: the fundamental aspirations of their profession for working with integrity to create high-quality care at least and often some sense of a better world.

However, the challenge for practitioners is in how to apply these faced with the complexities of service users and communities and the often contradictory expectations of their organizations. What can be confronting is being faced with a plethora of views and possible actions, and lacking a sense of clarity about which are ethically more acceptable. How do you balance the conflicting desires of family members in their different percep-tions of what dignity means or provide equal access to resources when these are severely limited? Alternatively, several possible courses of action can seem equally ethical, how do you then decide between them? Codes of ethics are also criticized for being culturally determined and too universal, a 'one-size-fits-all' approach (Briskman and Noble, 1999), and for not acknowledg-ing that there may well not be a 'right' answer. Because of this, the International Federation of Social Workers Code of Ethics states that its statement of ethical principles stays at the level of 'general principles' for practitioners to use in reflecting on dilemmas. In practice, Congress (2000) points out that practitioners often balance the code of ethics with the conse-quences of applying them.

Impact of challenges to integrity

Concern about how to engage with ethical or moral issues is demonstrated in an increase in the variety of literature related to ethical dilemmas and the impact on workers from what some writers name as 'moral distress' (Epstein and Delgado, 2010) or wrestling with issues of morality or integrity (Banks, 2008). Frequently, writers, like practitioners, give such examples as being expected to focus on throughput and outcomes as opposed to values and professional integrity (Banks, 2002). For Epstein and Delgado (2010, p. 9) moral distress 'occurs in the day-to-day setting and involves situations in which one acts against one's better judgment due to internal or external constraints'. They also suggest that unresolved moral distress can lead to a moral 'residue': 'the sum of the nicks in one's moral integrity and the self-punishment inflicted when one does not do the right thing', which can lead to withdrawal, conscientious objection or burnout. Similarly, a study of healthcare workers in psychiatric and elderly care units connects what they name as 'perceptions of conscience' with burnout (Gustafsson et al., 2010, p. 34) given that 'perceived lack of time to provide the care patients need and dealing with incompatible demands are burdensome and thus related to increased stress of conscience'.

Responding to ethical and moral dilemmas

In spite of the painfulness of such experiences, practitioners generally remain determined to practice in what they see as ethical ways. Banks, who interviewed senior practitioners in the social welfare field comments 'I was struck by the accounts that a few practitioners gave of their commitment to hold on to a set of deeply held professional values in the face of adversity or pressure' (Banks, 2010, pp. 2168–9). Writers generally agree about the confronting nature of such dilemmas and pressures, but there is less clarity about how to respond.

Possible strategies: individually and structurally

Epstein and Delgado (2010) emphasize strategies of being active about moral issues such as speaking up, building support networks, becoming involved in moral distress education and developing policies. This has similarities to Gustafsson et al.'s (2010, p. 35) suggestion of the value of:

> providing opportunities to learn to live with one's conscience through 'sharing' what one's conscience tells one, as well as other burdensome work experiences with coworkers and supervisors, (which) may increase

awareness of what constitutes reasonable demands and goals in daily
practice, which in turn may reduce stress of conscience and burnout.

From a nursing perspective Murray (2010) and Edmonson (2010) respond
to the prevalence of ethical dilemmas by advocating 'moral courage'. Murray
(2010, p. 2) contrasts moral arrogance: dismissing others ideas without
consideration with moral courage: 'commitment to stand up for/ act upon
one's ethical beliefs' in the face of adversity and personal risk. For some,
thinking about morality connects with spiritual and religious beliefs.
Edmonson (2010, p. 7) recommends a broader approach of creating a
professional culture than encourages moral courage to emerge though the
creation of 'sacred space, mentoring, peer support programs, and a partici-
pative leadership model', and generating knowledge about ethical theory
and decision making.

Linked to Epstein and Delgado's (2010) point about the need for policy
change, some writers and some codes of ethics indicate the value of engaging in broader structural change. The Canadian Nurses Association's (2008,
p. 5) code makes explicit the distinction between law and ethics; acknowledging that there 'may be situations in which nurses need to collaborate
with others to change a law or policy that is incompatible with ethical practice'. The writers also assert that 'the code can be a powerful political instru-
ment for nurses when they are concerned about being able to practice
ethically'.

Critical reflection and ethical issues

Some of these writers imply the value of opportunities to be critically
reflective: the desirability of exploring what moral distress or issues of
conscience are about in more detail and how to respond to them. Other
writers more explicitly link critical reflection and ethical or moral dilemmas. Valani (2009, p. 413) explores the dangers of unthinking 'moral
certainty', the desire to be confident that decisions made are 'right' without
reflecting critically on underlying values. She cites a particular example
related to a complex abortion issue (the pregnancy likely to end and risks
to the mother's health) where a group of nurses refused to be involved with
the termination. In concluding, she says that the nurses 'moral certainty
about the right course of action and seeming inability to reflect on alternate
values and actions challenges that they have done the work of moral
inquiry or even realized that reflection was part of their moral organization'. This links questions of meaning and values with the need for reflection or critical reflection theories to help manage the complexities of
practice.

Critical reflection theory and ethical complexities

Rolfe (2000, p. 4), for example, in considering integrity identifies a core issue of 'how to tackle the "one truth" argument of positivism without falling into the extreme relativism of the "no truth" argument advocated by some post-modernism'. He suggests what he calls a 'position which recognizes the futility of attempting to uncover a single truth, but which nevertheless argues that it is possible to commit oneself to a moral and epistemological stance with integrity and good faith. I attempt to argue, in effect, that although we can never be certain of what is true, we are still able to make choices'. The combining of postmodern and critical social theory in critical reflection also provides a way of managing this, seeing how to balance the diversity and flexibility of postmodernism with the expectation of socially just practice in critical social theory. Both approaches make explicit the influence of social expectations embedded in cultural norms. Critical social theory in critical reflection also reminds practitioners of the cultural and historical complexities of seeking 'truth': that what seems absolute to one generation of practitioners may be questioned by the next. Changing views related to adoption provide a good example of this with the change from past practice of forbidding further contact with birth families to current practice of positively encouraging it.

Using critical reflection can also enable practitioners to 'challenge, resist and remake the ways social structures play out in their lives' becoming more aware of assumptions in their practice that 'deny or devalue important personal characteristics in personal settings, leading people to feel that there is no room to incorporate their personal integrity into their work lives' (Fook and Askeland, 2006, p. 52). This then enables practitioners to act according to their values: in Rolfe's terms to make choices that come from a place of integrity and good faith. Similarly, the Canadian Nursing Association's Code of Ethics (2008, p. 37) suggests ethical reflection should begin with a review of the practitioner's own ethics and values, recognizing that there 'is room within the profession for disagreement among nurses about the relative weight of different ethical values and principles'. Implicit here is a postmodern acceptance of difference, which is then balanced with understanding of and engaging with discussion of values.

Edgar and Pattison (2011, p. 8) are also explicit about the need for reflection. They acknowledge the complexity of integrity and suggest that it is 'reflective capacity that we want to commend as the most important aspect of professional integrity in contemporary healthcare practice'. Reflective practice opens up the 'the development of a more intimate involvement of the moral-practical dimensions' (Sullivan, 1995). It is often in the process of being critically reflective that practitioners identify the sense of unease that often accompanies ethical dilemmas. Practitioners often described this as feeling uncomfortable or that something is just not sitting right. The process of reflecting critically about where this sense of discomfort is coming from encourages identifying the fundamental values and principles that the person prefers to operate from. It might be, for example, that a worker is reacting negatively to a colleague or service user, initially they make judgements about the other person – perhaps partly quite realistic ones. However, what becomes clear is that the underlying issue is something like: why do I not like this person when I believe I should value everyone?; or why do I think this person needs to do what I say/believe when I thought I believed in affirming diversity and difference? Having articulated the underlying ethical issue, the worker is then able to make an active choice about what they want to do: do they act from their preferred values and if so how can they best do that. Alternatively, if they decide that they will have to compromise or qualify those fundamental values, they must identify the costs and the best method of management.

The context of ethical issues

Critical reflection also helps with understanding the context of ethical dilemmas and being able to name these accordingly. Ethical dilemmas arise at various points of practice including and perhaps particularly in the difference between professional practice and organizational expectations – often expressed as the tension between desire for more holistic practice versus outcome focus. While this has always been the case to some degree, the tension is greater currently given a combination of economic stringencies. Most organizations in health and human services are wholly or partly funded by governments, so responsive to the expectations of their funding bodies and therefore influenced by political processes. Banks (2002, p. 34) provides a particularly telling example of this in interviewing a worker where are a service user has just committed suicide; her manager's first question is 'are the case notes up-to-date?' Baker also outlines the pressures on frontline workers after significant cuts to resources 'with even fewer options for supporting their service users, but with the same pressure to constantly "manage" risk' (Baker, 2013, p. 121). These issues lead to ethical dilemmas such as how much to advocate for a service user or a colleague or a policy, or about how much to put a different point of view, particularly one that might not be popular. Issues of fairness or justice are common ethical dilemmas related to organizational policies and practices.

Other ethical dilemmas relate to the interactions with and between other people and how practitioners should act towards them. Frequent examples here are conflicts between service users or colleagues or between a colleague and a supervisor. Such conflicts often leave the practitioner feeling caught or torn between opposing possibilities, often presented as dichotomies by the parties involved. Being critically reflective is helpful here in slowing down reactions, so that it is possible to identify the underlying values and influences to respond in a more nuanced way, moving beyond dichotomies.

There are also times when an ethical dilemma can be one that is shared across a group of staff. Critical reflection supervision groups can elicit these. One person's issue can generate discussion about how this particular issue is experienced as a more general dilemma or it can be that this specific issue is one that is shared. Sometimes the issue itself is not particularly large, but it symbolizes a general attitude or approach that feels or is considered to be an unethical or in some way unfair. This can be as simple as something like a particular group of service users or staff not being able to access organization resources such as a meeting room or a tea room. Alternatively, it can be more obviously significant such as the closure or restriction of a service or the application of a set of rules or guidelines in a way that disempowers a particular group.

In one organization, for example, one member of a critical reflection group raised the issue of being moved to another organizational site. This meant that service users had to travel further to access her service and for many of them this meant complicated public transport arrangements. At the same time, the organization had restricted access to organizational cars so that it was more difficult for her to be able to travel to service users. When she raised this issue and her feelings of anguish about what this meant, it quickly became clear that this was an issue that resonated with most of the others in the group. Once the particular issues that connected for this worker had been explored, the group as a whole identified what was common in their reactions. They expressed the kind of moral distress identified by Epstein and Delgado (2010): the moral residue of continually acting against what they believed was fair because of the organization's constraints. What was helpful was clarifying the underlying assumptions that seemed to differ between the organization and the practitioner's whose assumptions and values focused on:

- the accessibility of services for service users;
- the difficulties service users have due to their complex lives that made it difficult for them to attend appointments; and
- the challenges of a poor public transport service which places an unfair burden on service users.

They considered that the organization's underlying assumptions were:

- increased efficiency through minimizing administrative support is needed given budget; and
- colocating all staff offering the same service in one location is more important than dispersing staff to increase accessibility.

Individually, they had felt powerless to try to change what was happening and assumed that there was nothing they could do. When it became clear that this was a collective frustration, a different sense of energy developed and the group began to explore how they might raise this with management.

Examples of using critical reflection to engage with ethical issues

The following examples illustrate more specifically how critical reflection has been used in a variety of ethical dilemmas across a range of disciplines and practices. These include working with families, with others in organizations and in policy dilemmas.

Carol in community development

Background: Carol is a community worker employed by local government in a new, poorly resourced outer suburb of a large city. The community members also lack resources with high rates of unemployment and low incomes. Carol's role is to identify community needs and a community vision and work with interested community members on developing related activities. One of the needs identified early was for more activities for children and young people and a committee of volunteers was formed to develop an under 12 soccer team. This took quite some time, partly because of the requirements from the soccer league and fundraising for soccer uniforms, boots, and so on. During this time, Carol worked with the committee to identify how they wanted their soccer club to be. This essentially involved establishing ground rules such as: being actively inclusive (anyone from the local community would be welcomed, girls as well as boys, any cultural background); the emphasis was to be on teaching them to be 'good sports' (i.e., playing well and fairly, not 'hogging' the ball and not being too focused on winning) partly given the lack of experience of both the parents on the committee and the players.

Case study 7.1

Incident: A parent, Jack, always spent matches running round the ground shouting at his son Darran, telling him what he was doing wrong, that he was an idiot or worse. This particular week, he shouted several times 'don't be a girl'; several of the girls on the team and their parents were upset about this and complained to the coach. He also muttered loud racist comments about an indigenous player on the other team. Two parents expressed their concerned about the racist comments to a committee member, because their other children had heard and repeated them.

Carol's reaction: The issue of Jack's attitudes had come up previously at the committee meeting. Several parents/committee members were uncomfortable with how pushy they felt Jack was, but the general feeling had been that it was up to Jack; Darran was his son. Carol had felt uncomfortable with this partly from her own values of anti-oppressive practice and questioning when it was reasonable to challenge what felt like bullying attitudes at least to Darran. Her professional assumptions were in conflict: as a community worker was the most empowering thing to leave this to the committee to decide or ethically should she be taking a more active role in challenging such behaviour? Given the committee had already developed a culture of acceptance she decided to suggest they look at the issue implicitly using critical reflection to draw out assumptions and values.

Stage one

Given that the committee members were already individually and collectively agitated and concerned about the issue, it turned out to be relatively easy to suggest simply identifying all the different views about this and these were listed on a whiteboard. It was clear that everyone felt strongly though not necessarily in the same way. Many different views were expressed robustly. They included:

- Parents shouldn't hassle their kids like that and Darran hates it.
- Jack has a right to say what he likes to his own son.
- We don't want anyone putting the girls off.
- The girls play as well as the boys anyway, sometimes better.
- Kids need to learn not to pay attention to comments like that.
- We don't want an adult giving kids the idea it's all right to slang off like that.

- We want everyone to feel welcome at our club.
- I don't want people to make racist comments around here about my friends.
- It's not just about winning, we want the kids to learn about what's right and fair.

When the group looked at all the comments, one pointed out that the last one was where they had started as a group and that they had wanted to use being on the soccer team not only to play soccer but for their children to learn how to play well together, to be cooperative, respectful and resolve differences well. After more debate, there was general agreement about this and that they didn't want negative comments flying round about girls or boys or people from different cultures that reinforced old stereotypes. For Carol, this was a relief, essentially the committee was agreeing with her ethical position: not accepting racist or sexist attitudes that would undermine the team and by extension the community.

Stage two

Having agreed to what they thought in principle, the group were then faced with what to do. This generated even more discussion, with most people uncomfortable at the idea of talking to Jack, with some concerned about 'getting thumped'. Assumptions about conflict surfaced: that was hard or impossible to resolve or that it was best to walk away from it. In this situation, the committee felt they had talked themselves into having to do something: implicit in their clarity about values was the need to act. Eventually, the question was asked who could put this to Jack in the way he'd be most likely to hear it? Carol felt guiltily relieved that the assumption was it would be better coming from a male, given that Jack seemed dismissive of women. Finally, one suggested that it would come best from Jo, the coach who would be seen as the person in authority and traditionally as representing the club and the team's best interests. The coach was initially alarmed and reluctant, but as the group experimented with what to say and how to say it, he could see how to raise the issues with Jack in a way that was more likely to work.

Outcome: Jack did initially react negatively, but Jo persisted in explaining the background to the team and the committee's way of thinking. Jack left, making critical comments, but did come back with Darran the following week and just stood and watched. One of the committee members approached him for a general chat and over the next few weeks, Jack became more part of the support group for the team.

For Carol this reinforced using critical reflection to identify the issues collaboratively; power remained shared with her able to express views as an equal participant, although in practice, the committee articulated her dilemmas. She noted her reaction to who should talk to Jack (the logical extension of her concerns) and the contrast between her espoused theory: women can do this compared to her theory in action: relief when it was agreed Jo should as something to follow up in her own critical reflection supervision.

Policy issue in a health department: Pam's experience

Case study 7.2

Background: I work in a government health department that controls which drugs are available free to patients. I work in the evaluation section so don't usually have anything to do with decisions about which drugs are used, it is more to do with finance, other accountability issues and the results.

Experience: I was asked to write a memo in response to a health service (Service A) requesting funding for a particular high cost drug for two women awaiting cancer treatment. The drug is not usually funded because of the high cost, but the health service argued these women should have it for a short period because of delays in their treatment caused by a miscommunication with the service (Service B). Service B heard about the request and said that if it was funded they would request funding for 20 other adults not receiving the drug who could also benefit from it because of various complexities in them accessing treatment.

Why was this significant to me? I felt the memo needed to be seen in the context of the ethical issues it raised as well as process issues. For me, given there is limited funding in the health system, how do you decide who should get drugs that are possibly lifesaving? And who should make that decision? How can you balance out the miscommunication? Should that make any difference?

I also was being asked to take responsibility for something I didn't believe was my responsibility or my area's responsibility. I felt powerless, that I didn't know enough about it. I liaised with all the senior officers and got conflicting views, which caused a lot of tension. In the end the decision was made further up and I still had to write the memo, which I felt I didn't really agree with.

Stage one

When the group asked more about how she felt about the experience, Pam focused on her feelings of frustration about being asked to make a decision about something she thought she didn't know enough about. One group member asked: so if you had known everything about it, all the facts and information about what had happened with the communication, would you have felt better about making the decision? Pam found this a hard question to answer and in the end, concluded that she wouldn't, because if felt like a decision that had too many ethical issues. She also felt that she would be making a decision about how to spend public money, without the public having any idea about how their money was being allocated. She put the question back to the group: would you want to make this decision? Initially the group thought this was avoiding the issue, but it led to a discussion where Pam was asked again: so what really mattered to you about this? What's the most important thing? She responded that she felt she was being put in an impossible situation: there was no answer that everyone would be happy with. This was an aha moment: she added that's it, what's why it was so hard, I wanted everyone to be happy with the decision and it was obvious that that was impossible – unless money was no issue of course.

She then articulated that personally and professionally her underlying assumption or value was do what will keep everyone happy. This assumption contradicted other values of 'doing what is right'. It was clear to her that these were often not going to be compatible and given that she wanted to do the 'right' thing that she needed a new assumption about keeping everyone happy.

Stage two

For this group, the second stage happened two weeks later. Pam came to the session with a new assumption: I can't always keep everyone happy, which feels liberating. She had also been thinking about the complexities of 'doing the right thing' and wanted to explore the tensions between wanting to act ethically and how difficult it could be in principle to decide what this would mean. She concluded that what mattered was her intention to be right and having willingness to engage in inner or outer debate about the most ethical action so that she wasn't simply reacting. Her new assumption here was: maybe there is no right answer, but we need to have the debate.

When asked 'what difference would it make if you were faced with a similar situation?', she said that she would not have the tension of trying to keep everyone happy, and would also recognize that other people were likely to be working from their own desire to be ethical. She also acknowledged the complexity of the context: the competing groups wanting more healthcare funding and the question of whether funding should be limited and if so how. She decided to raise, in a policy meeting, the need for wider public debate about such issues. Primarily though, the lessening of tension came from seeing that sometimes there is no right answer, she decided she would remember this for other similar situations.

Whose responsibility is it? John's experience

Case study 7.3

Background: My organization was involved in developing a new programme – there was considerable political motivation to achieve certain outcomes within a set time. The programme advisors for the department funding the program suggested being careful about the timelines because a lot of factors were not in the control of the programme. This advice was disregarded and the outcomes and timelines were made public before the programme started.

Experience: The outcomes for the new programme weren't achieved and the programme manager, my colleague, was blamed for not implementing it quickly enough. He was publically blamed for this and placed under a lot of pressure to resign. In the same week, my organization launched its new values policy with emphasis on professional integrity. I didn't say anything at the time, I didn't know what to say.

Significance: I believe my colleague was unfairly blamed for the programme outcomes. The Department's advice, which clearly said the timelines were unrealistic, was ignored. I feel it has cast a shadow over his career and his skills and knowledge have been lost from my organization.

Stage one: group discussion

When asked more about what really bothered him about this experience, John said it was the hypocrisy of the organization: that they were publicly professing values of integrity when they had treated Frank so unfairly. His view was that the overall manager of the organization who had agreed to the timelines should have accepted responsibility and either resigned or resisted the pressure to have someone blamed. He asked how he could trust others in the organization or the processes and structures used as a result of what had happened. Due process had not been followed, so where was the justice for Frank?

After some discussion, which tended to go in circles as John reiterated his anger, a group member asked what this meant for John himself, how did he feel about remaining in the organization that he thought had treated Frank so badly? John struggled with this question initially, it was easy to name his anger towards the organization about Frank, and particularly to the overall manager, Jack, but he found it quite confronting to think about where that left him. He felt that implied in the question was a criticism that he had stayed. Reassured on that point, that is, the person asking the question said she was just curious having made a similar decision, he said that actually he did feel bad about staying, he felt that he was condoning the behaviour even though he had not been able to influence it and felt powerless to do so. He felt caught, he really liked working in the organization with the particular service user group and with the staff team he coordinated, but he felt guilty that he hadn't done more to support Frank. When asked to say more about that, he said he wished he had been more up front, stood up to the manager more publicly. Part of him had been afraid that he would also lose his job, which would have caused problems for him and his young family. However, when he was asked where he thought Frank was coming from, he said he was surprised that Frank accepted the decision, but that, in some ways, things had turned out well for him. He decided to travel, which he had always wanted to do and now worked in a field that suited him more. Frank reiterated though that wasn't the point from his perspective.

It seemed that this was a point of clarity for Frank, so he was asked a transition question: so where are you with this now? His response was: I'm feeling clear that for my own feeling of integrity, my assumption is I should have said more to support Frank.

Stage two

Frank began by exploring what his assumptions might be. He felt rather than new assumptions he needed to articulate more clearly and affirm old assumptions and values he hadn't been true to in this example. A first assumption was: 'my sense of integrity is important to me'; followed by: 'I want to be assertive about what I believe in'. When asked what he would do differently in a similar situation he said he would express his concern directly to the person in Jack's role, although he was concerned about how. This led to a discussion about strategies: how to express disagreement calmly and, where possible provide an alternative constructive suggestion. Frank acknowledged that of course he often had to do this in the workplace, so a third new assumption emerged: I know how to express my disagreement constructively; I can exert power in my workplace. Finally, Frank's view was that provided he expressed his views he would feel able to stay in the organization in a more positive spirit. He identified the phrase to reinforce his learning as: 'just say it'.

Summary

Ethical dilemmas are an inevitable aspect of professional practice, They can cause significant distress to practitioners with such consequences as disillusionment and burnout. Critical reflection processes provide opportunities to name such dilemmas, the feelings, thoughts and underlying assumptions and values connected with them. This often frees up thinking about how the dilemma is perceived in ways that enable the practitioner to either resolve or manage to live with the dilemmas.

Questions for reflection

- Think of an ethical dilemma you have experienced in your practice?
- What was your reaction? How did you feel? What thoughts did you have?
- What other perceptions could there be?
- How did you manage or resolve this? How does this sit with you?
- What support would you value for engaging with ethical dilemmas?
- How might you generate that support?

8 Managing Uncertainty, Change and Conflict

Uncertainty, change and conflict are inevitable aspects of organizational life. 'Professionals practice in an uncertain and ever-changing world and they need to develop creative, innovative and proactive approaches to professional practice (Titchen and Higgs 2002, p. 288). For many practitioners, the rate of change in organizations and society generally means they feel they are living with constant instability. Being critically reflective can enable practitioners to acknowledge their and their organization's assumptions and preferences about uncertainty and how to develop strategies to live with it. When uncertainty becomes specific change, practitioners will face different challenges and again being critically reflective encourages assumptions about change to surface, altering those that are unhelpful and developing strategies to work constructively with change – or to oppose it. Critical reflection enables people to unearth the values that are influencing their practice and Oliver and Keeping (2010, p. 103) suggest these can act as a 'beacon to guide us and help us make sense of challenges to our identity during times of change'. This chapter will also take further the issues in relation to conflict partly explored in Chapter 4, identifying how critical reflection can generate strategies for managing or resolving conflict.

Reactions to change

Organizational reactions

Organizational cultures have their own reactions to change, uncertainty and conflict and vary significantly, depending on the personalities of key individuals, past and current experience and the current organizational and social context. In an organization that had experienced three restructures in two years practitioners described the prevailing mood as 'just lacking in energy and motivation; it doesn't feel worth starting anything in case there is another change'. Understanding the context for organizational change is central to engaging constructively with it: what is happening globally, nationally, locally that might be influencing this change? Which factors can be influenced and when does a change need to be accepted and managed as well as it can be? Reactions will vary depending on what the change is and where it has come from: in an organization it will depend on whether the change is internally or externally driven and how those different drivers are perceived and understood. An external, politically driven change is more likely to be accepted if it benefits the organization and is congruent with organizational and individual values. Change that undermines cherished aspects of an organization or its capacity to achieve valued goals are more likely to be resisted. Sometimes, of course, resisting change can be valid: staff in one organization united to object to a proposed restructure that would have meant greater challenges to resources for service users.

Individual reactions

From an individual perspective, people will also react differently to change depending on whether the change comes from external forces or an internal shift and their own attitudes to and preferences about change. Some people simply have a personality that predisposes them to enjoy change, to find stability uninteresting and stagnating. For some this may be reinforced by past experiences of change that have led to improved conditions or a way of living out values more closely. Others will have varying degrees of comfort with change with some finding any kind of change unnerving or actively undermining. The resilience literature suggests that some individuals perhaps for genetic reasons combined with early life experience are more able to relish living with change and uncertainty or at least to see change as inevitable and an opportunity rather than a threat (McEwen, 2011). However, it also suggests that too much experience of negative change can become debilitating for most people. It is important then for each person in an organization to think about their own experience of and current reactions to uncertainty and change and the assumptions they make that will influence their reactions.

Petra worked with men who had abused their partners. She often felt angry about the men's behaviour and with some of them their apparent unwillingness to change. Her experience was of one of the men, Grant, saying that her attitude reinforced his negative feelings about himself, that he was not capable of being a better human being. When she explored this more

Practice example

deeply, she realized that her espoused values were in conflict with how she acted in practice: her belief from her religious tradition that everybody was of worth and could change versus the belief that some of the men she worked with were not capable of change. This clarified that she wanted to operate from her espoused belief and that she needed to make clear her anger was about abusive behaviour. This shifted her relationship with Grant and he began to react more positively.

How the change will impact organizations, teams and individuals will also influence how people respond. A key question is how can my, or my team's, sense of energy and organization be maintained in the midst of such change or as a result of change? Sometimes small teams feel quite separate from the broader organizational change. A sense of belonging and shared purpose in the team minimizes the impact of organizational change. When there is significant organizational change such as restructures involving loss of staff, people will be influenced by their own personal and social situation. Two people of the same age offered redundancy packages may react quite differently: one who is already thinking of retirement might respond enthusiastically; the other who expected to work for another 10 years, quite unhappily.

Reactions to change will also vary according to how the change has come about and the process used to introduce the change. Change is more likely to be accepted if people feel they have some degree of influence or choice – if it has been collaborative (developed with those affected by the change) or at least consultative (asking those affected about how they perceive the change) compared to change that is imposed (Auer, Repin and Roe, 1993). The pace of change also influences reactions to it. Slower paced change gives people time to adjust and adapt and allows for modifications if the initial plan isn't working. All of these, of course, have assumptions implicit in them and these are likely to be part of the organization's culture: the difference between an assumption of 'ground level staff have practice knowledge that needs to be taken into account' versus 'management are aware of the current economic and political imperatives and need to make the decisions'.

The challenges of uncertainty

It is also important to recognize the difference between uncertainty and change. Bridges (1991) identifies the potentially stressful period between some kind of change or the possibility of change being suggested and a decision being made and enacted. This period of 'transition' or 'in-between time' Bridges suggests is a time of disorientation and reorientation and it is important to acknowledge the anxiety that accompanies it. Whether the leader is a manager or a team member, Harle, Page and Ahmad (2010, p143) say 'a quality of effective leadership in turbulent and uncertain times refers to the capacity to hold onto the anxiety of 'not knowing', while enabling and retaining the capacity to act thoughtfully. This in-between time, which in spirituality literature is talked about as 'liminal space', is a time when a person may feel in a time of waiting, suspension, doubt and instability or insecurity, a time of standing on a threshold. For many people this in-between time is particularly stressful because it is not clear yet in which direction it is possible or desirable to move. It is particularly important to develop strategies that support staying in this in-between space for long enough to allow the development of clarity about how to move forward.

This time of simply having to wait is one that is often familiar to service users as well as to workers. An obvious example of this is waiting for a diagnosis related to an illness or the prognosis after an accident. There are also many examples of being in a period of doubt or indecision connected to relationships or being in a work position that is not satisfying. These raise questions of whether to seek change? Will things change? Will things get better? Is it just how I feel at the moment? Some people can feel quite immobilized by this in-between state; others find this so uncomfortable that they prefer to have any kind of decision rather than continuing to experience a sense of uncertainty. This partly relates to past experience: if a time of transition has been particularly painful or has ended badly, the impetus for finalizing a decision is likely to be greater. Being critically reflective can provide processes for recognizing the emotions and thoughts of this in between stage and how to manage waiting.

Once the change has been decided upon, there are then different challenges and again how these are mediated will depend partly on what meaning the person sees in the change. This will vary depending first how the change relates to the person's values: does the change reinforce or undermine values? Second, for many people coming to a decision brings with it a sense of relief. Now it is clear what the future will be and it is a matter of starting to act. There may still be a sense of loss even if there is also gain, the acceptance of the change also brings with it the letting go of what has been. Recognizing the grief that goes with change is an important aspect of being able to move on.

Practice example

A team who had been in an aesthetically pleasing building, where they were able to maintain contact with each other easily were moved to a larger building where they were in closer contact with the rest of the organization, but less connected as a team. While they could see some benefits of this move, they also regretted the loss of close contact and pleasant surroundings. It was helpful to acknowledge these regrets as a team so that they could engage more fully once they moved.

One of the strengths of the critically reflective process is that it encourages naming the feelings related to change that are uncomfortable. Simply naming these frequently enables practitioners to handle them more effectively: recognizing the need to sit with them, letting them go or using the process to reach a point of clarity for acting on them. Working through the process can also clarify the possibilities and choices for action. The second stage focuses on change, which may include attitudes, assumptions, strategies or processes. The expectation is that understanding will lead to change of some kind. Ferguson (2013, p. 91) suggests the process helps practitioners feel more empowered, to deal with the anxieties of practice that is 'confused and messy', when 'we can sometimes struggle to see a way forward or imagine the situation changing ... By becoming "unstuck" and being able to find ways of progressing through a difficult issue, practitioners are more easily able to find ways of progressing through a difficult issue'.

Practicing critical reflection enables those who prefer action to get better at staying in the moment, taking time to understand their own reactions and those of others in a particular context. This lessens the danger of acting too soon simply because of discomfort with uncertainty. It also allows time for articulating the underlying values and assumptions that are likely to be key to acting in what feels to be the most appropriate way. One practitioner, for example, commented 'I don't think it's my natural personality because I'm more of a problem solver ... so bringing it back and examining it all and doing the assumptions doesn't come naturally, but it's really beneficial' (Gardner and Taalman, 2013, p. 99).

As is hopefully obvious by now from the examples in this book, being critically reflective and/or more specifically using the two-stage critical reflection process also contributes to change both at an individual level and at the organization level. Practitioners become more confident in their own capacity to initiate change using constructive strategies for themselves, with colleagues in relation to the team, the organization and in seeking policy change. This is also change that is holistic for practitioners connecting life and work, being personal and professional. Fook and Askeland (2006, p. 49) from an analysis of evaluations from critical reflection workshops identify changes in people feeling more powerful: the reframing of power into different types – 'non-hierarchical, personal and emotional in ways that allowed them to feel more powerful and therefore to act in more powerful ways'. This is reinforced by Jasper (2011, p. 53) from using critically reflective writing in continuing professional development, with

> deeper reflective activity at this level, leading to practice change ... or even fundamental challenges to organizational culture ... As a result, the products of critical reflection are contributing to professional as well as personal development, whether at the level of the individual practitioner, within clinical environments or wider in terms of how practitioners are utilized and deployed within a service.

Hearne (2013, p. 139) who has used critical reflection extensively as a manager says being critically reflective 'has become integrated into how I approach life and work' and that 'I can say that I believe I can positively change how I feel at work. I can have hope about making positive changes at work that positively affect working relationships and bring about a better fit for myself and those with whom I work'.

Engaging with conflict

Conflict is inextricably linked to change and uncertainty. These often generate internal personal conflict with mixed feelings about what the change means to self and others, interpersonal conflict about different responses and conflict within the organization in various forms – between individuals and teams, between teams and managers and so on. Conflict can be creative and lead to new possibilities, but can also generate unhelpful vicious circles that make differences appear destructive (McLean, 2007, p. 333). These are influenced by the range of factors explored above as well as by the assumptions made individually and organizationally about conflict. Critically reflective practices can help break negative cycles of conflict and encourage more creative and open ways of operating.

Damien came from a family that had experienced many traumatic life changes. His response was to assume change would be damaging and to immediately embark on defending himself and/or his territory, in this example, his team. His team had mixed reactions to this: some felt he was jeopardizing the team's survival by being too combative, their assumption was it's better to keep quiet and hope you are forgotten about. Others valued his approach feeling he was ensuring the team's value was being upheld. These different perspectives eventually surfaced and Damien acknowledged that there was a middle ground of asserting the team's value.

Practice example

There are, of course, many situations of conflict that are experienced by practitioners: internal conflict as well as conflict between colleagues, in teams, with service users and supervisors. Reactions to conflict are influenced in similar ways to reactions to change and uncertainty. Assumptions about conflict reflect family, organizational and broader social and cultural beliefs. For some people, expressing conflict directly is assumed to be potentially destructive; for others conflict is what makes life interesting. These reflect differences in personality (VanSant, 2003) and being able to name these simply as differences is helpful in reframing conflict. White (2008, p. 179) points out that communication is complicated because of the attribution of meaning and belief:

> it is impossible for a family to hear what I say in exactly the way I intended it because their understanding will be mediated by the unique meanings and beliefs which they put upon it ... The worker must find ways to understand the 'sense' that the family make of their own situation ... (especially in the context of differences of gender, race, culture and belief).

The same comment could be made about workers in organizations: conflict is often influenced by lack of understanding of where the other is coming from.

Managing rather than resolving conflict

An important difference in approach to conflict is that between managing and resolving conflict. Some conflict cannot be resolved, reaching agreement is simply not possible given the differences in values and preferences expressed, the question is how to accept differences and work with them. Postmodern thinking reinforces that there are many ways not one way. This can lead to reframing conflict as exploring and valuing difference rather than another person seeking to impose a view on another. Asking 'how else might this situation or experience be seen?' allows new points of view to emerge accepting that there are many ways/perspectives not just one. This often connects to a postmodern moving beyond binaries, being stuck in a 'right/wrong, your way/my way' tension. If there are many perspectives or possibilities, it is somehow easier to accept that the other person has simply chosen differently.

> Dan and Ray (case managers in disability services) had been in conflict for various reasons over the two years they had worked in the same team. Usually these conflicts were about minor things: Ray not being on time, Dan arguing about how case notes were written for joint service users: Ray saw Dan as pedantic and Dan saw Ray as 'slack'. Eventually this came to a head and their supervisor asked them both to go to a workshop on working with difference. They were astonished by the framework presented, which seemed to outline their conflicts so clearly and named them as simply differences in personality and approach. This took the heat out of their arguments and they were better able to negotiate compromises.
>
> **Practice example**

Critical reflection and change, uncertainty and conflict

Critical reflection also reminds people about their fundamental values, which can provide a sense of certainty and stability when everything else seems in flux. Discussion about these enables people to see what is common as well as what is different. For example, two workers may be operating from the same underlying values of commitment to achieving the best service for their service users, but they may not agree about the most effective approach. Connecting at the level of values can move people to appreciate the intent of the other and so to be more open to what the other has to suggest. The experience of mental health workers using critical reflection in supervision was that they developed more collaborative relationships: 'being more aware of others' perspectives and how they might differ from one's own generated deeper, shared understanding and contrary, to what might be expected, greater capacity to work together' (Gardner, 2013, p. 75).

Being critically reflective also enables practitioners to stand back from the immediate to look more broadly at what is happening and what is influencing their reaction both individually and as part of the broader organization or community. Identifying what is happening in the broader social context can help to put a particular conflict into perspective: while it still may not be perceived as desirable, at least it may feel less targeted and personal. This may also help with seeing what possible directions there may be and how to clarify the issues that will affect these. Standing back from the immediate can also include exploring your own reaction: how much is this reaction to do with approaching conflict in general, how much is it to do with this particular conflict? This can of course, mean that you see something more clearly and want to do something about it. Baker (2013, p. 116) points out there is a 'dangerous' side to critical reflection in that you can find yourself in conflict with the organization in an unexpected way and then have to decide what to do about this especially 'when we realise that solutions to our dilemmas are not always readily forthcoming'.

Examples of using critical reflection with change, uncertainty and conflict

The following case studies use critical reflection to generate different perspectives on managing uncertainty, change and conflict. The first relates to an income security organization concerned about an impending policy change about eligibility for a particular benefit. The second example is from a worker faced with managing uncertainty. The third is related to a drug and alcohol focused organization where there is conflict between service users and between practitioners.

Managing change: income security team

Case study 8.1

Background: An income security team was faced with a national government decision about changes to a benefit. Essentially this meant that the benefit would be less available than it had been and that people with a range of disabilities would need to be assessed more regularly to see whether they should be seeking paid employment. Many of the staff felt outraged by this change. They knew that many of their service users would be affected and would experience further hardships in lives that were already challenging. They also felt that this was a politically motivated decision with politicians wanting to be seen to be tough on people who were misusing benefits. From their experience in the field, the workers believed that there were very few people, particularly people with disabilities, who were in this category and that the new changes would do considerable harm and achieve little in preventing benefit abuse.

The managers of the programme in a particular office decided to see whether approaching this as a group using a critical reflection framework would enable the group to engage with this change in some more constructive way. The group agreed to try this although there was some degree of scepticism about whether anything would be achieved.

Stage one: exploring the issue

The session began with the manager outlining the changes suggested, then the workshop facilitator provided an outline of critical reflection theory and processes. This was followed by small group discussion about people's reactions and exploration of where those reactions were coming from particularly the assumptions and values that people felt were being compromised.

What emerged from this was initially the identification of how people felt – a mixture of anger, frustration, powerlessness and a sense of futility. Many workers felt torn between a desire to simply leave in protest versus a fear of not being able to find other work versus a desire to try to change things – perhaps to refuse either explicitly or by avoidance to comply with the new policy.

Some of the underlying values and assumptions that were identified were:

- I shouldn't support unfair policy.
- People with disabilities should not be unfairly targeted.
- I don't want to let down my service-user group.
- I can't do anything to change this.
- I feel as powerless as the people that I'm working with.
- I can't maintain my sense of integrity and support this policy.

As the group looked down at this developing list on the whiteboard, they expressed relief about the sense of common values that was clearly emerging. They also appreciated the sharing of internal conflict about how to approach this new policy. This led to an exploration of how people managed the inevitable conflicts that were part of working in this organization. Many participants gave examples of other ways that they felt conflicted about organization policy. This generated a change in mood within the group from a sense of hopelessness about seeking any kind of change in the policy to a recognition that they had previously found ways to manage policies that they felt were disempowering for their service users. They also acknowledged that they had been assuming that their service users would be powerless in relation to these changes. While this was certainly true for some, others had been involved in action and advocacy groups that could influence policy. Sometimes service users could act more freely and powerfully than workers.

Some new, more hopeful assumptions emerged:

- it is possible to bring about change in this organization
- change can come from inside and outside pressures
- we have knowledge about how to manage organizational systems that will be lost if we simply leave
- we can express our disagreement about policies and actively seek change
- part of our role is to advocate for our service users.

Stage two: moving toward change

The workers returned to small groups and spent some time clarifying individual assumptions and values and how these were shared or different in their small groups. The results of these were then shared across the groups and at this stage it became clear that there was a significant degree of agreement. This included:

- Advocacy for our service users is a primary part of our role.
- We can assert when we believe that our service users are genuinely unable to work.

- We need to convey to individuals and families our belief that people are generally honest rather than an attitude of looking for dishonesty.
- Integrity is about having done our best, not necessarily about 'winning'.
- We can seek system change through coordination and collaboration.
- Service users can also be powerful in seeking change.

Having worked out these underlying assumptions and values, the group was able to move to a position of seeing how they could generate shared activity. Two gave an example of a previous policy where their team had documented specific case studies where people had been disadvantaged by how a different benefit was implemented. They had used these case studies to build a case for changing the process of administering the benefit, which resolved the problem. This reinforced the sense of possibilities for change and action in the group and agreement was developed about how to manage and coordinate information about the impact of implementation of the new policy. The senior managers also agreed to raise concerns with the senior management team with the aim of influencing how the policy would be presented.

Dealing with uncertainty: Peter's experience

Case study 8.2

Background: I have been working as a district nurse based at a community health service for seven years. I really like this kind of nursing, I love supporting people in their own homes and also like being based at community health – I was in a hospital setting previously, but a community-based health service seems to fit better with district nursing.

I'd been vaguely aware of organizations in the local area manoeuvring for more influence over the past year but hadn't really paid a lot of attention, until six months ago the local hospital – a major health provider in this area, commissioned a report about changing how health services are coordinated, and the report recommended district nursing be combined and all fit under the hospital system.

Experience: I raised this with my line manager in community health because I still hadn't heard anything more and she confirmed that this was still being talked about, but nothing had been decided. I got really angry with her, close to shouting at her and I felt terrible about it afterwards and apologized, but I still feel bad, which is why I've brought it up.

Beginning significance: I've never done anything like that in supervision before, have had disagreements but always seen them just as that. It feels really out of character for me and it's made me realize I am more upset about this possible change than I realized.

Stage one

When Peter explored this experience more, he identified his surprise at his anger, and that he anger was not really directed at his supervisor, it was feeling angry with being left in limbo, feeling unsure whether the change would happen and if it did what it would mean for him. He also felt somewhat undermined by the process, the lack of consultation and access to information. This felt very rational, rather than reflecting on emotions, so he was asked again so what is it that *really* bothers you about this, he unearthed that being uncertain made him feel that he wasn't valued, his assumption was that being left in limbo mean that you weren't important enough to bother about.

When the group idea stormed what else might be happening that meant no decision had been made, they identified a range of issues: conflict among the organizations and wrestling between senior managers about where services should be located; political uncertainties about funding; the criticisms the government had had about other suggested changes that might make them reluctant to embark on more. Peter agreed that all these made sense and that this helped make the impact of the uncertainty feel less personal. One of the group then asked, so why do you think it affected you so strongly? Peter then connected this experience to his experience as a child of his family moving constantly because his father had trouble keeping a job. This meant the family lived with uncertainty and Peter felt his views/feelings about wanting to stay, to be settled somewhere were never seen as important. Making this connection personal, he reflected, helped him see why his anger was so strong. He could also see that his assumption was that you just have to put up with uncertainty, you can't do anything about it.

Another group member felt concerned that this link to family issues was undermining a perception of Peter's right to be consulted. She expressed this and Peter responded that he felt differently: recognizing where the strength of his anger was coming from enabled him to see what was happening at work more realistically. He could recognize the other factors likely to be influencing what was happening, but thought he had a right to be consulted and informed. He also now felt he could raise these issues more appropriately with his supervisor.

Stage two

Peter was now able to articulate what he thought were more constructive assumptions:

- Uncertainty is not necessarily personal.
- It's reasonable to expect to be informed and consulted about changes that will impact on my role.
- I can develop strategies for managing uncertainty more positively.

The group then asked how these assumptions would change what Peter did. He decided he would first raise with this supervisor his desire to be informed and consulted about any change that related to his work area; he would also raise this with other team members and suggest strategies to increase mutual support given the stress of the uncertainty. He also thought he would use the first assumption to remind himself that the uncertainty was not related to his sense of worth. Peter decided to use the phrase: 'uncertainty is part of life' to remind himself about his learning form the reflection.

Managing conflict: Sarah's experience

Background: I was the coordinator of a mental health team in a city suburb. One of the workers in my team, John, had been working with a long-term service user, Jess, for several months. Jess had requested a referral to a withdrawal unit to change her drug use, including the reduction of anxiety related drugs.

Specific experience: John was advised that a place was available and organized for Jess to be admitted. The day before she was due to go, John was told that another service user had been admitted that had a history of conflict with Jess. The unit had decided Jess would have to wait. John told Jess she couldn't go and why. Jess felt John was blaming her for the conflict with the other service user and refused to work with him anymore. I then had to work with Jess when I was feeling overwhelmed with other work.

Why this felt significant to me: I found this all very frustrating, but particularly having to pick up John's work when I was so busy. I thought he should have been able to give Jess the message in a way that meant she would keep on working with him.

Stage one

Initially, Sarah continued to express her frustration about John and gave other examples of when she has found him hard to work with. Eventually the facilitator asked her to concentrate on this example as the group was finding it hard to focus on what the key issues were. One group member then asked so what was it that was really frustrating to you? Sarah answered it was John, his inability to work with Jess. The group member then asked so what about Jess's conflict with the other service user how did you feel about that? Sarah responded that she hadn't really thought about that, but then added that Jess often ended up in conflict with other people. When the group then, at Sarah's request, idea stormed where John might have been coming from a strong theme that emerged was maybe John wanted to challenge Jess on the impact of her continuing conflicts. Perhaps John would be frustrated that Sarah had agreed to work with Jess rather than expecting or supporting Jess to work out these issues with John.

Sarah felt quite challenged by this, but acknowledged that in retrospect this made a lot of sense and that she hadn't given John an opportunity to say what had happened from his perspective. She also realized that she hadn't thought about the part that the unit played in this: why had they decided at the last minute that they couldn't take Jess. Her assumption had been 'I have to respond and take responsibility for everything'; 'I have to pick up the pieces and calm things down if there is conflict'. This was an 'ouch' moment for Sarah, she reflected that in her family of origin, it was the role of the women in the family to 'keep the peace' at all costs, which reflected their culture and history.

Stage two

Sarah's recognition of these underlying and deeply held assumptions immediately precipitated her wanting to explore changing them. The group idea stormed some possibilities and what emerged were two new main assumptions: 'sometimes conflict is productive and needs to be allowed to happen' and 'responsibility can be shared, I don't have to take it all'. From these new assumptions, Sarah thought that it wasn't too late to work on this particular situation. She decided to meet with John and explore how he felt about what had happened and see whether he was prepared to work with Jess again. Depending on how this went, she would meet with John and Jess and make explicit to Jess the need to work to manage conflict/differences. Third, she decided to contact the unit to discuss how decisions were made about allocation and timing and suggest some changes. The phrase she chose to remind herself of this new learning was: 'whose issue is this?'

Summary

Change, uncertainty and conflict are inevitable aspects of professional practice, each with its particular challenges influenced by personal and professional experience and the organizational and broader social and political context. Critically reflective practice can create change, uncertainty and conflict, but also generates ways to manage these: to acknowledge the emotions involved and constructively engage in processes for accepting and affirming difference in a way that can lead to more collaborative practice.

- How do you currently feel about change, uncertainty and conflict? What are your assumptions about each of these?

Questions for reflection

- Where do those feelings and assumptions come from? What are they influenced by?
- Use an example from your own experience to explore whether those assumptions and your values are helpful in relation to change, uncertainty and conflict or how you would want to change them.

9 Interprofessionalism and Critical Reflection

Being able to work constructively and actively with a range of other professional disciplines is an expectation of practice for most workers. The quality of practice, in a variety of settings, depends on recognizing and valuing what each discipline brings. This needs to happen across disciplines as well as between organizations and both can be challenging. One of the benefits of being critically reflective is that it is increasingly seen as part of professional practice across many disciplines. With common training and agreement about how critical reflection is understood, staff from a wide range of disciplines can use critical reflection as a common language. The process of critical reflection can also help with identifying different professional assumptions and what these might mean for effective team work. Specific examples from healthcare organizations will be used here to illustrate how being critically reflective can engender mutual understanding and lead to changed work practices.

The changing nature of interdisciplinary practice

There is a long history in health and human services of efforts to encourage professional disciplines to work together within and between organizations, not always with success. The language used has changed over the years to reflect changes in thinking. Scott (1993, p. 1) writing about child protection found: 'Exhortations to organizations to work together have become well-worn and well-meaning clichés, particularly in the wake of inquiries into the non-accidental deaths of children yet the goal of inter-organization collaboration often remains elusive.' In 1998 Ray advocated the move from what was then called a multidisciplinary model: 'professionals operating in individual silos with limited communication between them' to interdisciplinary practice, which 'requires common values, a common vision, and an intuitive understanding of teamwork' (p. 1374). Levine et al. (1994) talk about multi- and interdisciplinary practice but also stress the importance of partnerships between organizations and communities. The idea of 'case management' was to develop a more effective and coordinated way of providing services across organizations and disciplines (Payne, 1997; Guransky, Harvey and Kennedy, 2003) with practitioners across disciplines taking on essentially the same roles.

Crawford indicates there are now many terms used to suggest more collaborative ways of working (2012). What is more often named as the 'interprofessional' agenda examines practice across disciplines both within and between organizations. Different language includes 'integrated' or 'joined-up' practice or case management where there are systematic ways of ensuring that professional skills and knowledge are provided in coordinated and collaborative ways. Sometimes this approach has focused on competencies in practice so the question becomes who can do this, rather than assuming a particular discipline should. However, this has been criticized for being too pragmatic and not including the indefinable aspects of practice: Sturgeon (2010) points out the dangers of 'McDonaldisation' becoming too specific about how particular goals are demonstrated such as requesting nurses to always demonstrate caring in the same way rather than responding intuitively and sensitively to what is needed at the time.

Key influences on interprofessional practice

Organizational responses, to the impetus for greater interprofessional collaboration have varied. Some of the challenges were identified in Chapter 4: the tendency for organizations to be funded for narrowly defined fields of practice, for example. Some of the key influences are the extent and quality of relationships, the role of place and space and service user perspectives.

Extent and quality of relationships

Individual professionals are also influenced by their own experiences of working with others from different professions. For some this has been challenging and conflict ridden; for others a rewarding and enriching process and again this can reflect organization culture. Hickson (2013) found mixed views in social workers she interviewed with some feeling challenged by the differences between professions. Often what helps the process is taking time to build positive relationships across disciplines both within and between organizations. This may happen informally and is often maintained by informal contact, but it does help to have formal processes endorsed by managers. Saunders (1990, p. 5) points out that 'Each team member may also have to deal with personal stereotyping and work out with the team how such type-casting is best used, or if necessary, overcome.' Some organizations have also developed strategies to balance the sense of divided loyalties that individuals may experience. In some large health organizations, for example, each staff member has a discipline specific clinical supervisor and a line manager who can be from any discipline. This can provide a useful balance between shared professional understanding and learning across disciplines.

There have been many initiatives both at organizational and government policy levels to encourage greater flexibility and cooperation across disciplines and organizations. One recent example from Australia is YP4 initiated by four medium-sized non-government organizations as a model of 'joined-up' practice for young people experiencing both homelessness and unemployment. The aim was to develop partnerships with other service providers including mental health, drug and alcohol, housing and employment by building relationships across organizations to ensure better coordinated and more holistic service delivery. Feedback from the YP4 case managers supported the view that 'meeting service user need is often predicated on the extent and quality of interorganization relationships'. In practice, the case managers were primarily focused on forming personal and pragmatic relationships that would benefit service users rather than being formally defined or inflexible (Grace, Coventry and Battenham, 2012, p. 147).

Rachel, a psychiatric nurse, and Jake, an occupational therapist, both worked as case managers in an organization for people with disabilities. In a critical reflection group, Rachel identified her fear that she would lose her specialist knowledge and skills because she wasn't using them much. Jake agreed and after Rachel's specific experience was explored, the group turned to the issue of specialist versus generalist. They identified all the aspects of their roles in common and were surprised how many there were. However, they also identified some specific specialist knowledge useful to be aware of so that they could use each other as 'consultants' as needed. The list was written up and each worker kept a copy for future reference. When they revisited this issue six months later, the shared view was that they now valued and used each other's specific expertise more effectively and that this had somehow freed them to more fully appreciate what was shared.

Practice example

The role of place and space

The role of place and space can also be significant in an organization, helping or hindering interdisciplinary processes. These include where an integrated team is located, how physically easy it is for people to build relationships and be able to communicate, how pleasant the environment is as a place to work. Again in YP4, Grace and Coventry (2010) looked at co-location as a specific strategy in encouraging integration of service delivery. Workers from a housing organization were located with the national income security organization in a regional office. Before the co-location, workers at each organization expressed concern about impact on service users and service identity and distinctiveness. However, the findings confirmed benefits including 'greater respect and trust between professionals from different backgrounds and with different status ... informal information exchange, learning and sharing ... enhanced feelings of teamwork and belonging ... improved morale among staff; and enhanced communication, learning and understanding of roles' (Grace and Coventry, 2010, p. 170).

Service user perspectives

Part of the complexity of interprofessional practice is the range of perspectives that need to be taken in to account: the service user, which may be individuals, groups and/or communities; the mix of professionals (individually and collectively); the organization/s and the broader community; and political interests. Most or all of these will interact with each other in a given context.

The service user perspective is generally seen as central in this. Service users tend to want a more holistic approach including all aspects of their personal wellbeing. They have also been critical of the lack of information sharing and coordination in their care within and between organizations, commenting that communication between team members is lacking which may be detrimental. From a service-user perspective, being involved in health and human services often means connecting across many disciplines and/or organizations. This is particularly obvious in something like chronic illness, where an individual might need specialist input from a physiotherapist, an occupational therapist and a social worker as well as continuing contact from their general practitioner and a specialist related to their specific illness. Equally, an individual, family or community concerned about issues related to death and dying could be connected to palliative care nurses, a specialist palliative care doctor, social workers, bereavement workers, a pastoral care/spirituality workers and/or psychologists as well as volunteers. The array can be bewildering, how, from a lay perspective, do you become clear about who does what? Service users also comment on the sheer numbers of people they are managing and coordinating, which can feel overwhelming. This is especially so given there is often a degree of overlap. In palliative care, for example, Stanworth (2002) argues that you could legitimately see 'spiritual care' as an aspect of practice for many disciplines. This view is supported by Rumbold (2003) who suggests responsibility for spiritual care is shared by the whole team, with leadership by specialists such as pastoral care workers. The questions then are: When or how this is made clear to service users? and How do they participate in information sharing and decision making?

Crawford suggests that a more active sense of consumer rights 'have, and continue to, push forward interprofessional collaborative working' (2012, p. 39) with service users as partners in the process. However, in the disability field, Marks (2008, p. 67) argues '(a)ll too often, interprofessional rivalries, hierarchies, different professional languages may prevent working together to the detriment of service users'. Recognition of this has led to increased expectations of professionals valuing what each other does and using their respective skills and knowledge to resource service users and communities. Ideally, then decision making is at least shared if not made by service users and communities themselves. What can be challenging is remembering to include the service user as a valued member of the decision-making team given the pressures of internal organization issues and structures. Service users have considerable agreement about what they want from service providers. These include putting the quality of the relationship first, demonstrating being human as well as having skills and knowledge (Croft and Beresford, 2008, p. 393), which is likely to apply across all service providers. The move to people with disabilities having greater control over how funds are spent on their access to services reflects their desire to be treated with respect and seen as knowledgeable about their own health and wellbeing. This will also orient services differently to hearing the service user's voice as primary. Thinking about what will best meet the preferences of the service user/community reinforces the importance of effective interdisciplinary practice.

The impetus for working across disciplines and organizations may be to increase access to services particularly in areas that are seen as having less access or being 'underserved'. This can be either geographically or related to a specific issue. Levine et al. (1994) found that in such communities a 'community–academic health centre partnership' worked best where the community were involved in the partnership and led and owned particular programmes combined with interdisciplinary practice and training of indigenous community health workers. Other organizations have allocated one or a small group of staff to particular geographic areas to provide a range of services to individuals and/or the community. This allows them to understand more deeply the networks between individuals and to work with community connections rather than undermining them (Gardner, 2006).

Ellen worked in an organization funded to provide a range of services across a large geographic area. She was allocated to a particular local government area and began by meeting other service providers and the service users already known in the area. She found that she could respond to most issues herself, requesting 'consultation' or supervision from other specialist staff as needed. Over time, she could also see how she could link people together for mutual benefit: a woman with a disability with another who felt isolated. She began to work with community groups interested in a more community development approach, aiming to strengthen community relationships. Service users and community members commented how much better it felt to be responding to one person who knew the community rather than 'a cast of thousands' making flying visits.

Practice example

What do professions share and what is distinctive?

Such views prompt discussion about what professional disciplines share and what is distinctive. Each profession has tended to emphasize what is distinctive in order to assert its worth. How important are the boundaries between professions? To what degree are they permeable? Are there dangers of losing what is distinctive in interprofessional practice? Barrett, Sellman and Thomas (2005) identified 14 professions from teaching to occupational therapy to police in the United Kingdom. Generally, the professions endorsed the value of interprofessional practice, identifying benefits for service users and communities where professionals were able to understand each other's roles and how they could be shared. However, their reactions varied depending on how the concept had been introduced and managed. There were some concerns about the erosion of particular philosophical approaches and skills: for example, Oliver and Pitt (2005, p. 182) suggest that youth workers are more likely to be successful interprofessional workers if they gain 'more confidence about what they have to offer in terms of their skills, knowledge and practice'. Those who had always worked in an integrated model were more likely to see the benefits for themselves and those they worked with. These discussions are complicated by the differences of perception within professions about their role and purpose, debates about how professional values should be expressed in practice; as Thomas (2005, p. 193) says 'clarity cannot always be achieved'. Postmodern theory as outlined in Chapter 2 reinforces that individuals as well as groups will have different perceptions depending on a particular context and how dominant ways of thinking are expressed. Managing the uncertainties this generates as well as those discussed in the previous chapter becomes then part of managing interprofessional practice.

Combining professional and interprofessional identities

Connected to engaging with these issues is the question of identity: do we see ourselves as what we do or do we do a particular role because of who we are? Oliver and Keeping (2010, p. 102) suggest that 'the very idea of "identity" is in a state of flux, owing to the constant and ongoing change that is challenging the central structure of our social world'. They use the idea of occupational rather than professional identity to focus on the activities of professionals rather than identity as status. For some workers, there is a sense of loss about being in a generic team where all are named as case managers carrying out essentially the same roles although their initial professional training may be quite different. Part of what is challenging for professionals is the kind of role blurring identified in Chapter 4: what Oliver and Keeping (2010, p. 90) name as 'the overlap of roles and the perceived encroachment of traditional territory (which) can lead to practitioners questioning their place within the interprofessional system'. Not everyone sees this as an issue, of course, those who are used to working with other disciplines may see it as less of an issue.

Managing to balance professional and interprofessional identity rather than seeing these in opposition seems to help. Clouder et al. (2012, p. 464) explored the impact of being a peer facilitator on (inter)professional identity and concluded that having 'a sound sense of one's own professional identity, or as one student put it "understanding where you're coming from", is important for openness to interprofessional engagement in an interprofessional teaching and learning environment'. They suggest conceptualizing 'the interprofessional self as a face of professional identity'. This fits with feedback from students about the need to develop understanding of their chosen profession in order to better value the benefits of interprofessional practice (Chipchase et al., 2012). However, others would argue that the skills of being interprofessional need to be taught at the same time as being professional: 'a climate of reflexive awareness of our own personal motivations and identifications is necessary so that we retain the positive aspects of our own different professional identities while understanding and addressing any unhelpful and obstructive aspects in our relations with other professional groups' (Oliver and Keeping, 2010, p. 101).

How critical reflection fosters interprofessional practice

So what generally helps with interprofessional practice? A common theme here is the need for some kind of systematic reflective practice or critical reflection, particularly in exploring and valuing difference. One of Hickson's (2013) interviewees pointed out that learning to be reflective is important in multidisciplinary teams enabling all team members to understand the job and organizational context and the differences in professional orientation.

Scott (2005, p. 140) suggests it is important to recognize that trying to work more collaboratively is likely to generate conflict at organization and individual levels and that 'collaboration requires the effective management of conflict'. This may be at inter- or intraorganizational level, interprofessional, inter- or intrapersonal and strategies need to fit each level. Conflict partly comes from attitudes embedded in professional training that has traditionally emphasized differences; tertiary education is generally provided in silos like those of the professions in the workplace. Miers (2010, p. 76) suggests '[p]rofessional education is not just a process of gaining knowledge and skills, it is a process of socialization into the vales and characteristics of a professional group'. However, there are signs of this changing. Professional training is now more likely to prepare professionals to work together. While this varies significantly there are more examples of courses sharing something like a common first year or an interdisciplinary subject that encourages understanding of different roles.

The value of being critically reflective for interprofessional practice is also seen as providing a shared understanding from a common theory base and so a collective language. For many disciplines, critical reflection can provide a common language for exploring practice when the language of their disciplines is significantly different and the jargon related to the discipline quite inhibiting to understanding each other. Wilhelmsson et al. (2012) suggest the value of identifying mutual components of professional competence including reflection and critical thinking and a shared language. Training across disciplines in critical reflection gives a shared set of theoretical approaches that cross professional boundaries. Such training can begin in tertiary training courses and continue or be developed in practice. This also contributes to having a language for sharing perspectives.

Given that 'the complexity of interprofessional practice is not only about skills, knowledge and theory, but very importantly is hinged on professional values' (Crawford, 2012, p. 163) a key benefit of critical reflection identified by professionals is being able to see where there is common ground across disciplines, particularly shared values about approaches to practice in general.

As part of a shared way of thinking, critical reflection also reminds workers to think about the broader social context and how it is influencing their particular field of practice. As Pollard, Thomas and Miers (2010, p. 4) identify reflection is important given

> the implementation of interprofessional working within health and social care is not isolated from wider social influences. Factors which affect society as a whole also affect the way that individuals working within the health and social care services operate in relation to their own roles, to colleagues from other disciplines and to service users.

Ideas about occupational or professional identify are also influenced by the social context: by public perceptions of doctors or social workers or teachers in turn influenced by media sensations as well as the sharing of community and individual narratives.

Barrett and Keeping (2005) affirm that what fosters interprofessional practice is knowledge of professional roles with clarity about what is shared and what is distinctive, being willing to participate, confidence about your own role and a sense of competence in it, and being able to communicate openly, with trust and mutual respect. They add that shared power also helps, acknowledging the inevitability of conflict and the value of setting ground rules that try to minimize it. They also identify reflection and supervision as helpful strategies. Having critically reflective supervision embedded in the organizational structure is often mentioned as a useful aspect of interprofessional practice although it has its own dilemmas. Fronek et al. (2009) explored boundary issues in interprofessional practice with over 100 health professionals including occupational and speech therapists, social workers, nurses and doctors. They concluded that critical reflection was essential in managing professional boundary issues given the wide range of educational backgrounds, skill and experience. Feedback from participants supported the value of interprofessional training 'and the ability of those participants to learn from each other' and '[m]any participants saw the practice of supervision and peer support as a concrete strategy they could introduce into their workplace' (Fronek et al., 2009, p. 24). They concluded '[a] supervision model suitable for interdisciplinary teams needs consideration and would also require clinical managers to be knowledgeable in professional boundaries and process oriented supervision that moves beyond administrative supervision' (Fronek et al., 2009, p. 26).

One of the challenges of interprofessional practice, Miers (2010, p. 83) suggests, is the 'lack of shared understanding of established support roles for learning'. Hickson (2013) interviewed four social work managers about their role in creating a reflective culture; two were managers of multi-disciplinary teams in healthcare and two were managers in a federal government organization. 'These social workers saw their roles as providing leadership in reflective practice given their relative limits of power; influencing both new social workers and experienced social workers to be reflective. In addition, these managers saw themselves as the organization's champion for reflective practice, attempting to introduce a reflective framework for all staff. They saw this as producing and developing workers who were flexible, able to adapt to changing situations and willing to learn from their experiences. These managers suggested that, in reality, all workers are interested in evaluating their work and learning from their mistakes, but argued that social workers take it further by examining assumptions and deconstructing their practice' (Hickson, 2013, p. 148). The use of interdisciplinary supervision groups is an obvious response to this allowing cross fertilization across disciplines and structures that support being critically reflective. Critically reflective supervision including peer and group supervision has been explored in detail in Chapter 6. The value of formal critical reflection for interprofessional supervision groups has been clearly demonstrated across a range of health and human services (Fook and Gardner, 2013). The unearthing of basic assumptions, which can be generating conflict in interprofessional teams, is part of the critically reflective process, for example, between those assuming the individual is at fault and those who assume the system is causing the individual's problems. Identifying these can help each person see that their assumptions are overly simplistic and to develop a greater and hopefully shared complexity. Critical reflection individually or in supervision groups can also be a place to explore issues of conflict, identifying other perspectives and possible sources of action as identified in the previous chapter.

Examples of using critical reflection in interprofessional practice

The following are practice examples of how critical reflection has been used in interprofessional practice – a large healthcare organization using supervision to increase interprofessional practice, an individual feeling challenged by differences in professional practice and the experience of palliative care services in developing training in spirituality/pastoral care across disciplines.

Southern Health: a health care organization using critical reflection in supervision across allied health disciplines

Case study 9.1

The Southern Health experience demonstrates an organizational initiative to encourage greater interdisciplinary practice through the development and implementation of supervision across disciplines. Southern Health is a large metropolitan health service with over 400 professionals in Allied Health Continuing Care (full and part time). The project was initially developed with a panel of senior clinical staff and discipline-based managers, including the allied health director and a project manager, Eddie Taalman, an occupational therapist. The allied health area had nine professional groupings: physiotherapy, occupational therapy, speech pathology, social work, psychology, dietetics, podiatry, music therapy and exercise physiology. When the project began, how supervision was organized and perceived varied significantly across disciplines, some had developed formalized supervision practices, but others had no supervision. The project group decided on two days of training in supervision and critical reflection for staff groups of 20 to 25 at a time. These groups had practitioners from across the organization, so there could be some from the same team but not necessarily. Once staff had completed the training, they were allocated to interprofessional peer supervision groups to meet on a regular basis using critical reflection.

Initially, some of the groups were concerned about being allocated to an interprofessional group, particularly where they might not know the other staff. Some workers had positive experiences of being supervised by someone from a different discipline saying that this often gave them a usefully different perspective. Others had found this less helpful and missed the particular orientation of their discipline and this influenced their attitudes towards the supervision group. Reactions also varied depending on how much staff were already working together in a more integrated way. Some were in teams they described as basically doing the same work with some specialization whereas others describe their team as a group of specialists working together.

Each training group was offered a follow-up session at least six months after their initial training. Before the session, the groups were asked if there any particular issues that they wanted to explore and the session began with these. Most of the groups felt there were many advantages in the interdisciplinary nature of the supervision groups. It had taken time to establish the culture of the group so that all group members felt comfortable with talking about experiences they felt challenged by. Most of the groups were keen to use the session to practice critical reflection having become clearer about what they had not understood in the initial training. They did, however, comment that the theory and process of critical reflection provided a common approach across disciplines, which was helpful in bridging their philosophical or practice differences. Sharing specific experiences in the group also illuminated how each discipline would approach a particular situation and how this might be misconstrued by those from another discipline.

These initial findings were supported by a more in-depth evaluation with a particular team – the rehabilitation in the home team (RITH). Focus groups with team members identified that 'a particular change in practice was changed attitudes to other disciplines in general, as well as more specifically to those in the critical reflection group'. This partly came from seeing the other disciplines experience similar feelings and challenges, and thus feeling less 'threatened' by them. The experience of belonging to the supervision groups generally meant developing 'respect and rapport' for and with other disciplines' (Gardner and Taalman, 2013, p. 100). Participants also identified feeling greater openness to difference, which made it easier to approach others, including those from other disciplines about complex or difficult issues in the workplace. Those in two of the focus groups distinguished between what they did in supervision groups as part of critical reflection and what happened in case management or case discussion. They considered that in critical reflection they explored their general approach to work rather than discipline-related strategies about treating a specific condition. One person, for example, said:

it's not so much about how a physio does their work, or a nurse does their work, or how I do my work, maybe it's how I might respond to somebody, because we have discussed things to take into account personal and professional relationships and what that means. And just listening to the themes that arise you find there is a commonality between the whole lot of us. (Gardner and Taalman, 2013, p. 101)

The findings from the Southern Health experience suggests the value of embedding critical reflection in supervision groups as part of organizational structures as a way of reinforcing or of developing interprofessional practice.

Note: this example been written up in more detail in Gardner and Taalman (2013).

Individual perceptions of difference across disciplines: Brenda's experience

Case study 9.2

Brenda was the only social worker in a critical reflection group in a small rural hospital, which also had three nurses, an occupational therapist and physiotherapist. The group had been meeting every six weeks for a year, for an hour each time.

Background: I am the only social worker in a small rural hospital. I had been seeing a service user, John, who was dying. He had no family locally, he had few friends left alive and those were not mobile. He really would have preferred to be left alone to die at home, but this wasn't seen as acceptable in the community, partly because he lived in an old shack with no heating or cooling. He had requested in writing that he not be revived or given medical treatment to prolong life.

Specific experience: I went to see John just to see how he was and whether he needed any social work support. It seemed to me that he was close to dying, but I wasn't sure, I hadn't seen anyone as close to death before. I also wasn't sure if he was in pain from the noises he was making and he couldn't communicate verbally. I asked Kate the nurse on duty to come and check on him and she said there was really nothing that could be done for him. I had a feeling he was going to die soon, so I stayed. I thought he shouldn't be on his own and Kate obviously wasn't going to do it. Then I was again worried he was in pain, so I asked her to come again. She was quite dismissive, so I went back and sat with him. Suddenly, an alarm went off on the monitor and Kate rushed in followed by the other medical staff and they started trying to revive him. I tried to tell them that he didn't want to be revived but they just ignored me and I went away.

Why was this significant to me? I feel quite upset even writing about this again. John had wanted a peaceful death, not to have his life prolonged – not that that reviving him worked, he died anyway. I felt really frustrated with Kate that she had been so dismissive when I wanted her to check he was alright, but she then paid attention and did what he didn't want. I also felt completely ignored and powerless – like John I suppose.

Stage one

Brenda started by saying she still felt the mix of frustration, sadness, indignation, humiliation that she felt at the time of the experience. Sheer frustration was what she felt was strongest at John not getting what he wanted and her not feeling heard. 'Banging my head against a brick wall is what it felt like.' The parallels she said were clear, neither she nor John felt heard, they were both powerless in the system. She also felt this was typical of her role: she'd been put in a box of the wishy washy, touchy feely social worker compared to the practical nurses and doctors. When asked when else she felt like that, she said often in case management meetings where she often seemed to be the one asking how people felt about something and what they (the service user) wanted.

Initially in the discussion, Brenda needed to vent her feelings of anger. She found it hard to identify her own assumptions, and eventually said she couldn't imagine ever feeling she understood where Kate was coming from, so it would be useful to idea storm this, which elicited the following:

- I should be keeping people alive by doing whatever I can.
- People don't really want to die before they have to even if they thought they did ahead of time.
- Dying is scary, I don't want to sit with someone who is dying.

- I don't like just waiting round, not knowing what's happening.
- Social workers are more comfortable with feelings, they can sit with someone.
- Other staff/the community will expect me to do whatever I can to keep this person alive.
- I don't like this patient, he's always grumpy, I don't know how to relate to him. Social workers can talk to anyone.

Brenda was surprised by this list, and it helped her identify how different some of her assumptions were:

- People have a right to die how and when they want to.
- People have a right to not be resuscitated.
- Social workers are good with feelings, uncertainty, people, just sitting with whatever happens, but can also be practical and act sensibly.
- Dying is scary when you don't know what to expect.
- Nurses should know what to expect when people are dying.
- Nurses should be comfortable with people who are dying.

One of the nurses in the supervision group pointed out that the different assumptions Brenda and Kate were making reflected not only tensions between professions but between individual professionals and community views. There was general agreement about this and the challenging nature of these issues.

The facilitator brought the focus back to Brenda, asking so how are you seeing this now? Brenda responded that she felt both validated in what she had to offer as a social worker and more aware of the dilemmas that she and Kate might have shared. This led on to the second stage.

Stage two

Brenda thought that in retrospect she had assumed other professionals would or should see things the same way she did. She was surprised how many 'shoulds' she had for Kate. She also now felt that she had assumed reactions to her as a social worker as opposed to a nurse that were not necessarily the case and that social workers and nurses would always react differently. Two new assumptions developed from this: were 'what I have to offer as a social worker is valuable, I want to keep the touchy-feelys' but also 'I need to check where other professionals are coming from' instead of making assumptions. Thinking about the community context had reminded her that there are many views about death and dying. She affirmed her belief that John should be able to decide on his own death, but acknowledged the need for community education to change attitudes more broadly. She also wondered about suggesting training for all the staff about death and dying. Strategically, she decided to raise these issues at appropriate times with individual staff with the aim of getting the organization to develop community education sessions. Finally she decided her prompt would be 'where are we each coming from?'

Pastoral Care Networks Project: training across disciplines

Case study 9.3

The experience of the Pastoral Care Networks Project is a good example of a team using an interprofessional approach. This project aimed to increase access to pastoral/spiritual care for those who were dying and their families in two regions in Victoria, Australia. The project approached palliative care teams in local areas to ask first whether they thought there was a need for training in pastoral/spiritual care in the area. Almost all of the staff agreed that there was such a need and suggested that training be developed for them as the staff group as well as for the volunteers involved in their programmes. The staff varied depending on the geographic area but generally included a doctor, palliative care nurses, district nurses, a social worker and/or a psychologist and/or a bereavement worker, pastoral care worker or chaplain (either paid or voluntary) as well as palliative care volunteers. There was ready agreement across all of the sites that everyone needed to be involved in training and that it would be advantageous to have the team trained together, paid staff as well as volunteers. The reasons for this were partly that pastoral/spiritual care was something that teams thought everyone needed to be aware of and able to respond to. People pointed out that it was difficult to predict who a particular patient or family member would choose to talk to. It was often in the process of carrying out a particular task that someone would choose to raise issues that they were finding confronting. It didn't always seem appropriate to say wait and I will ask the pastoral care person to come and see you; and sometimes even if this suggestion was made the patient would be reluctant to agree. Because of this, the teams felt that they all needed to be better at responding, and able to recognize when they needed to refer on to a specialist pastoral care worker or chaplain.

As a result of these conversations, a three-day training programme was developed. It emphasized an experiential and reflective approach to learning, understanding the influence of social context and practicing skills in pastoral/spiritual care. When the training was evaluated, one of the significant benefits identified was that members of the team felt that they knew each other better and the similarities and differences in their roles more clearly. A typical comment was: 'Very important to have the education as people have so many different ideas – good to exchange ideas so don't get set into our own little pattern'. The general feedback reinforced the value of the interprofessional team and the ability to see what could be shared and what was distinctive.

Summary

Expectations have increased that professionals will work in interprofessional teams within and across organizations. Some find this challenging, undermining a sense of professional identity; more often professionals value the learning that comes from other disciplines, provided their own discipline remains valued. Service users and communities also benefit from shared and coordinated practice. Being critically reflective enables professionals to identify the similarities in underlying values and assumptions and to develop a shared language and theory base for a shared understanding of practice.

Questions for reflection

- What has been your experience of working with other disciplines?
- How have you reacted to this? What have you valued? What have you found challenging? What do you see as shared assumptions and values and what if any are distinctive?
- What do you think can make interprofessional practice more effective?

10 Embedding Critical Reflection in Individual and Organizational Practice

These can be daunting times for practitioners in health and human services. Expectations are high: professional training emphasizes holistic and high-quality practice. Practitioners are generally extremely motivated to contribute to the wellbeing of individuals and communities, to act as agents of change according to their own and the values of their professional discipline. However, they are confronted with considerable challenges: the current economic and political climate, which stresses outcomes rather than processes, the increasing complexity of the issues individuals, families and communities are facing and the uncertainties of constant change, combined with expectations to move towards interprofessional practice. The organizations where practitioners are based have their own sets of issues to manage: the pressures of less income combined with greater expectations including the creation of learning cultures, demonstrating effectiveness according to what may be experienced as sometimes inappropriate funding strategies and managing practitioners overwhelmed by levels of change and uncertainty. The organizational culture will reflect these and some cultures are better than others at retaining a climate of supporting workers whatever the prevailing context.

These pressures generate a range of tensions in practice often experienced as the differences between the expectations of how things 'should' be compared to how they are or how I can work, compared to how I would like to. Some of these are experienced as ethical or moral dilemmas: struggles to respond to complex situations, which may reflect the lack of resources, what are experienced as unjust rules or simply many different preferences where it seems impossible to find the 'right' way forward. These tensions combined with the busyness of practice can contribute to interpersonal and intra- and interorganizational conflicts, which again add to the stresses of practice. All of these can lead to practitioners questioning their practice and sometimes their commitment to it. A sense of powerlessness can undermine practitioners' capacity to act to resolve or at least engage with such issues to determine how to manage them.

Practicing holistically and with integrity

What this book has done is to suggest that being critically reflective can provide a way of approaching practice that enables practitioners to manage their practice more effectively, while retaining a sense of integrity about it. Langston Hughes, an African American poet and social activist kept hope and dreams alive even in times of despair as expressed in his poetry (Hughes, 1994, p. 32). The aim, in being critically reflective, is to keep alive the dreams of holistic, life affirming practice. Without this, what practitioners describe as their fundamental values or feeling of integrity is compromised which can lead to negativity, moral distress or residue. This is not to suggest that being critically reflective can possibly resolve all of these issues or avoid having to compromise or simply accept what can't be changed, but rather that it can engender a way of being that is more sustaining, enabling and empowering. With this way of being, it is clearer when and how to seek change.

The theories and processes of critical reflection validate the holistic approach of professional practice, but also provide the complexity of ideas needed to engage with what Schön (1983) called the 'messiness' of practice. The practitioners interviewed by Hickson (2013) reinforced the value of understanding and actively using the underlying theories of critical reflection, embedding them in reflective processes. The combination of theories reinforces holding together apparently opposing perspectives in a way that leads to new meaning. This might mean, for example, balancing the postmodern expectation that there are always many ways to see any issue and the critical social theory expectation of seeking social justice. Alternatively, it might be validating subjectivity as well as questioning perspectives given the influence of context and history. Awareness of the concept of binaries from postmodern thinking contributes to seeing how your assumptions from using reflective practice tend to either/or ways of practicing.

The holistic aspect of being critically reflective validates the inclusion of the whole of the person, for practitioners as well as those they work with. Actively working with emotions as an important source of information and should be included in learning along with thoughts and physical reactions, assumptions and values. This means seeing the interconnectedness of the personal and the professional, how for each person, the personal and professional are intertwined and can influence and inform the other. Being critically reflective fosters understanding the influence of personal and social history on professional practice, how each person is formed by where they have come from as well as their current social context. Articulating this helps with deciding to what degree past beliefs, assumptions and values are accepted, modified or relinquished and new ones affirmed. Accepting spirituality is a related aspect of holistic practice, recognizing the centrality of what is meaningful in a subjective sense for each individual, which may or may not include religious beliefs. Recognizing all of these in the self, compels seeing that others have their own equally valid subjectivity and to value such diversity. This subjectivity is balanced by expectations of ethical conduct, including a socially just approach and understanding of the influence of the broader historical and social context.

Embedding being critically reflective in practice

What then more specifically does being critically reflective mean? Essentially, this means including a critically reflective attitude to all of practice, whatever kind of work you do in any organizational context. To be critically reflective is to develop a critically reflective attitude to life, or particularly here, to work in general, rather than seeing critical reflection as purely something that you do. Having such an attitude can permeate all of practice, how you perceive and engage with change, uncertainty and conflict, with ethical issues and organizational contexts. What is clear from the range of examples used in the book is that critical reflection is a theoretical approach and a process that can be used across disciplines to foster effective individual and interprofessional practice. Issues covered have also demonstrated the range possible – from issues with individuals and families, with work teams, the practical, relational and policy aspects of organizational life, with their related ethical and other conflicts. The aim is for a critically reflective approach to simply be part of how you respond. In any situation then, the theories of critical reflection would be influential; the processes of exploration and questioning would happen naturally. It might be, for example, that a colleague catches you in the passageway and asks for advice. Rather than automatically responding with answers, you would be more likely to ask some key questions: Where are you coming from? What else might be happening? How else could this be perceived? This would mean the issue is considered more deeply rather than simply being reacted to. Similarly, in work with service users, in organizational or community meetings, you would be more likely to ask about underlying assumptions. Of course, how you do this is important and needs to reflect the culture of critical reflection. You might in a community meeting, for example, say 'I wonder if we are all feeling frustrated because we are taking for granted there is nothing we can do to change this?' or to a service user, 'What do you think has got you thinking this way?' or 'How does what other people think about this affect you?' Depending on who you are talking to you might translate the language, rather than talking about assumptions, you might ask so where do you think that idea comes from or what seems important to you about this?

Partly because it is a holistic approach to practice, being critically reflective also encourages self-care. It validates paying attention to all of yourself in your context as well as to those you work with in theirs. Being critically reflective means having more awareness of how you are feeling, what you are thinking, how you are reacting and what is influencing these. This is particularly helpful when you are wrestling with ethical dilemmas or 'moral distress' issues that confront fundamental values. Creating the capacity for an inner reflective space fosters picking up more quickly when you are stressed, exhausted, angry, upset or in any way needing to pay attention to your own wellbeing. It also enables you to question why you are feeling or thinking that way, what patterns or assumptions you are tapping into and how you might need to change these. Actively using the underlying theories of being critically reflective also legitimizes taking into account your own 'subjectivity', recognizing how your own values interact with professional values in your reactions to practice.

Developing your own ways of being critically reflective

Being critically reflective does need to be learnt. How you develop this capacity will, of course, depend on you: your own preferred learning style, your personality, your personal and professional background and the context in which you practice. As the theory of critical reflection asserts there is no 'one right way'. This means it is important to remain aware of what you need to sustain a critically reflective approach, what particular combination of time and activities will work for you. Depending on your organizational context and culture, these may all fit within your workplace. Alternatively, you may need to be active about ensuring that your needs are met in a combination of internal and external strategies. These are only limited by your creativity. You can build critical reflection into your life in various ways: deciding to use time while you are driving to or from work or on the train or bus, asking your supervisor/supervisee to use a critical reflection approach, building in journaling in the morning before it's busy or at the end of the day when it's quiet, agreeing to meet for a critically reflective lunch/coffee with a colleague, participating in a critically reflective supervision group and so on. It is a matter of working out what balance of formal and informal processes will work at this point, and reviewing this regularly. The time used here is balanced by time saved from wasted energy agonizing over specific issues and in having to fix the consequences of rushed decisions.

The culture and challenges of being critically reflective

Specific processes for doing critical reflection were outlined in Chapter 3 and most of the following chapters end with examples of experiences of using critical reflection. These demonstrate some of the range of issues raised in, and challenges of, critical reflection. One of these is willingness to be vulnerable, to 'put yourself on the line', acknowledging that there is an aspect of your practice that you don't fully understand or that you feel actively unhappy with. Developing a culture or climate of critical reflection enables individuals to feel more comfortable exploring a particular experience with another person or a group. Working with others clarifies that, at a fundamental level, workers often share more values and assumptions than they expect: belief in the worth of their service users, hope for positive change and desire to improve the lives of those they work with. Sharing at the deeper level implicit in critical reflection enables workers to understand more clearly where they are each coming from and this in turn means they are generally more able to work effectively together. Trying out the processes of critical reflection usually leads to a greater sense of comfort about using them.

Issues of vulnerability and choice

Given this vulnerability, if an organization is implementing critical reflection, there is debate about whether participation should be voluntary and it is preferable to create a culture in which people want to come to critical reflection training and/or supervision. Ideally, of course, organizations involve their staff members in the decision of whether to implement critical reflection training and processes, so that it is a shared and consensual decision. Sometimes, critical reflection is initiated by those on the ground, but then needs also to be accepted by those more senior, so that critically reflective practices are not marginalized. It can also help if those implementing the decision are explicit about why they think the training is valuable and what they expect to happen as a result. There are benefits in organizations formally endorsing critically reflective practice (Reynolds and Vince, 2004; Gardner and Taalman, 2103) and in structures that foster critical reflection such as individual and peer group supervision. Funding is needed to support implementation of critically reflective practice first for initial training, then ideally for training for new staff, review and evaluation sessions for existing staff.

However, even when staff are involved and the organization endorses critical reflection, some may still feel there is not enough choice about participation. Rather than focusing on the binary of voluntary versus involuntary, it is more helpful to think about a continuum of voluntary/involuntary that allows for the complexity of mixed feelings about this. Sometimes people are fearful of trying anything new, particularly where there is a degree of vulnerability and it is easier simply to put it off, justified by pressure of work. Some resent being told something is compulsory on principle and others are wary of the rationale behind involuntary training. Where participating in training is compulsory, it can help to allow space for practitioners to express their views. Usually, by the end of the training nearly all are committed to trying the process. Reinforcing the group work principles of getting to know each other first and starting with less challenging experiences reassures most of these participants. In continuing critical reflection groups, some people simply need more time to observe the process in the group before they feel comfortable with participating. The changing nature of some groups is challenging, where new members come into established groups. On the other hand, if there is a core of experienced members, the process is likely to be so established that new members will join in more easily. It helps to remember that each time someone leaves or a new person arrives the group culture will shift and group members may need to time to rebuild trust. Refresher sessions – a reminder of the underlying theory and processes, particularly group culture, can help.

However, in my experience, there are a very few workers who remain unwilling or unable at a particular time to become critically reflective. They may feel too new and vulnerable professionally and/or currently experiencing a range of personal and professional issues. For a combination of reasons, they may not feel able to expose themselves to the process, particularly in a group that is new to them. For some people, it is more appropriate to start critical reflection in a one-to-one relationship where there is already trust – in individual supervision or with a critical friend, or for the person to try the process on their own. It is of course also fair to say that some people more easily embark on being critically reflective. Some people would say that they have always been reflective or critically reflective, but haven't had the language to name this as such. Others would say they struggle with the process: they find it hard to access their feelings or underlying assumptions and values.

Expectations of change

An expectation of change or of being able to act is also a central aspect of being critically reflective. Again the examples provided throughout, show how individuals use the process to change something internally: affirming existing assumptions and values or changing to more enabling assumptions and/or to change something externally, to act differently in ways that alter relationships, develop new activities or strategies. Some would say that their internal changes lead to external changes in team or organizational culture. Groups using critical reflection also demonstrate the possibilities of change: shifts in mutual understanding, joint seeking of new policies and processes and initiating activities within and external to their organizations.

Finally...

Finally, being critically reflective suggests that life is interdependent. Individuals influence and are in turn influenced by those they work with, the organizations in which they are based and the prevailing culture. The theory and processes provide ways of remaining resilient within the inevitable uncertainties, conflicts and dilemmas of professional practice.

At its best, being critically reflective is about creating or allowing an open inner and outer space, which holds opposites together in a creative tension. Like the liminal space of spirituality, it encourages standing on the threshold of the new, but waiting for clarity before taking action. In what can feel like a more mystical or sacred space, emotion, intuition and dreams have equal validity with the rational and thoughtful, they co-exist so that differences can inspire creativity that is life affirming, what Sneed (2010) calls 'human flourishing'. It is holding together opposing ways of thinking and feeling, seeing the world and allowing these to be so that something other can emerge, that affirms the values of holistic and socially just practice.

Bibliography

Allan, L. (2013) 'Thinking critically about student supervision', in J. Fook and F. Gardner (Eds) *Critical Reflection in Context Applications in Health and Social Care* (London and New York: Routledge), pp. 105–16.

Anderson, L.L. (2012) 'Inner and outer life at work: The roots and horizon of psycho-analytically informed work life research', *Forum: Qualitative Social Research*, 13(3) Retrieved from http://0-search.proquest.com.alpha2.latrobe.edu.au/docview/1086921213?accountid=

Argyris, C. and Schön, D.A. (1996) *Organizational Learning 11: Theory, Method and Practice* (Reading, MA: Addison-Wesley).

Armstrong, D. (2004) 'Emotions in organizations: disturbance or intelligence', in C. Huffington, D. Armstrong, W. Halton, L. Hoyle and J. Pooley. (Eds) *Working Below the Surface: The Emotional Life of Contemporary Organizations* (London: Karnac), pp. 11–27.

Armstrong, D. and Huffington, C. (2004) 'Introduction', in C. Huffington, D. Armstrong, W. Halton, L. Hoyle and J. Pooley. (Eds) *Working Below the Surface: The Emotional Life of Contemporary Organizations* (London: Karnac), pp. 1–10.

Auer, J., Repin, Y. and Roe, M. (1993) *Just Change: The Cost-Conscious Manager's Toolkit.* (Adelaide: South Australian Health Commission).

Bager-Charleson, S. (2010) *Reflective Practice in Counselling and Psychotherapy* (Exeter: Sage).

Baker, J.G. (2013) '*Cringe*-ical reflection? Notes on critical reflection and team supervision in a statutory setting', in J. Fook and F. Gardner (Eds) *Critical Reflection in Context Applications in Health and Social Care* (London and New York: Routledge), pp. 117–26.

Baldwin, M. (2004) 'Critical reflection: opportunities and threats to professional learning and service development in social work organizations', in N. Gould and M. Baldwin (Eds) *Social Work, Critical Reflection and the Learning Organization* (Aldershot, UK: Ashgate), pp. 41–55.

Banks, S. (2002) 'Professional values and accountabilities', in R. Adams, L. Dominelli and M. Payne (Eds) *Critical Practice in Social Work* (New York: Palgrave).

Banks, S. (2008) 'Critical commentary: social work ethics', *British Journal of Social Work*, 38, 1238–49.

Banks, S. (2010) 'Integrity in professional life: issues of conduct, commitment and capacity', *British Journal of Social Work*, 40, 2168–84.

Barak, M., Travis, D., Pyun, H. and Xie, B. (2009) 'The impact of supervision on worker outcomes: a meta-analysis', *The Social Service Review*, 83(1), 3–32.

Barrett, G. and Keeping, C. (2005) 'The processes required for effective interprofessional working', in G. Barrett, D. Sellman and J. Thomas (Eds) *Interprofessional Working in Health and Social Care* (New York: Palgrave Macmillan), pp. 18–31.

Barrett, G., Sellman, D. and Thomas, J. (2005) *Interprofessional Working in Health and Social Care Professional Perspectives* (Houndmills: Palgrave).

Berry, T. (2009) *The Sacred Universe Earth, Spirituality and Religion in the Twenty-First Century* (New York: Columbia University Press).

Bishop, V. (1998) *Clinical Supervision in Practice* (Houndmills: Macmillan).

Bolton, G. (2001) *Reflective Practice Writing and professional development* (London and Thousand Oaks: Paul Chapman and Sage).

Bond, M. and Holland, S. (1998) *Skills of Clinical Supervision for Nurses* (Buckingham, Philadelphia: Open University Press).

Boud, D. (2010) 'Relocating reflection in the context of practice', in H. Bradbury, N. Frost, S. Kilminster and M. Zukas (Eds) *Beyond Reflective Practice New Approaches to Professional Lifelong Learning* (London: Routledge), pp. 25–36.

Boud, D.J., Cressey, P. and Docherty, P. (2006) *Productive Reflection at Work: Learning for Changing Organizations* (Routledge, London).

Boud, D. and Solomon, N. (2003) '"I don't think I am a learner": acts of naming learners at work', *Journal of Workplace Learning*, 15(7–8), 326–31.

Bridges, W. (1991) *Managing Transitions Making the Most of Change* (Reading, MA: Addison-Wesley).

Briskman, L. and Noble, C. (1999) 'Social work ethics: embracing diversity?', in B. Pease and J. Fook (Eds) *Transforming Social Work Practice* (St. Leonards, NSW: Routledge).

Brookfield, S.D. (2000) 'Transformative Learning as Ideology Critique', in J. Mezirow (Ed.) *Learning as Transformation* (San Francisco: Jossey-Bass), pp. 125–48.

Brookfield, S. D. (2005) *The Power of Critical Theory Liberating Adult Learning and Teaching* (San Francisco: Jossey-Bass).

Brown, A. and Bourne, I. (1995) *The Social Work Supervisor: Supervision in Community, Day Care and Residential Settings* (Buckingham: Open University Press).

Brown, D.R. and Harvey, D. (2006) *An Experiential Approach to Organization Development*, 7th edn (New Jersey: Pearson/Prentice Hall).

Burchell, H. (2010) 'Poetic expression and poetic form in practitioner research', *Educational Action Research*, 18(3), 389–400.

Canadian Nurses Association (2008) http://www.cna-aiic.ca/sitecore%20modules/web/~/media/cna/page%20content/pdf%20fr/2013/09/05/18/05/code_of_ethics_2008_e.pdf#search=%22moral%20code%22

Canda, E.R. and Furman, L.D. (2010) *Spiritual Diversity in Social Work Practice the Heart of Helping* 2nd edn (Oxford: Oxford University Press).

Carroll, M. (2010) 'Supervision: critical reflection for transformational learning (Part 2)', *The Clinical Supervisor*, 29, 1–19.

Chipchase, L., Allen, S., Eley, D., McAllister, L. and Strong, J. (2012) 'Interprofessonal supervision in an intercultural context: A qualitative study', *Journal of Interprofessional Care*, 26, 465–71.

Clouder, D.L., Davies, B., Sams, M. and McFarland, L. (2012) '"Understanding where you're coming from": discovering an (inter)professional identity through becoming a peer facilitator', *Journal of Interprofessional Care*, 26, 459–64.

Cohn, E.S., Schell, A.B.B. and Crepacu, E.B. (2010) 'Occupational therapy as reflective practice', in N. Lyons (Ed.) *Handbook of Reflection and Reflective Inquiry* (New York: Springer), pp. 131–58.

Compton-Hall, M. (2003) '"Not all people are like me" addressing diversity from a newfound awareness', *Teacher Education and Practice*, 16, 143–55.

Congress, E. (2000) 'What social workers should know about ethics: understanding and resolving practice dilemmas', *Advances in Social Work*, 1(1), 1–23.

Coulshed, V. and Mullender, A. (2001) *Management in Social Work*, 2nd edn (Houndmills: Palgrave).

Cranton, P. and Taylor, E.W. (2012) 'Transformative learning theory seeking a more unified theory', in E.W. Taylor and P. Cranton (Eds) *The Handbook of Transformative Learning Theory, Research and Practice* (San Francisco: Jossey-Bass), pp. 3–20.

Crawford, K. (2012) *Interprofessional Collaboration in Social Work Practice* (London: Sage).

Cressey, M., Boud, D. and Docherty, P. (2006) 'The emergence of productive reflection', in D. Boud, M. Cressey and P. Docherty (Eds) *Productive Reflection at Work* (London and New York: Routledge), pp. 11–26.

Croft, S. and Beresford, P. (2008) 'Service users' perspectives', in M. Davies (Ed.) *The Blackwell Companion to Social Work*, 3rd edn (Oxford: Blackwell), pp. 393–401.

Crowe, M.T. and O'Malley, J. (2006) 'Teaching critical reflection skills for advanced mental health nursing practice: a deconstructive-reconstructive approach', *Journal of Advanced Nursing*, 56(1), 79–87.

Delaney, C. and Watkin, D. (2009) 'A study of critical reflection in health professional education: learning where others are coming from', *Advances in Health Sciences Education*, 14, 411–29.

Dewey, J. (1934) *Art as Experience* (New York: Capricorn Books).

Dirks, J.M. (2012) 'Nurturing soul work: a Jungian approach to transformative learning', in E. Taylor and P. Cranton, *The Handbook of Transformative Learning Theory Research and Practice* (San Francisco: Jossey-Bass), pp. 16–130.

Driscoll, J. (2000) *Practising Clinical Supervision* (London: Balliere Tindall, Harcourt).

Edgar, A. and Pattison, S. (2011) 'Integrity and the moral complexity of professional practice', *Nursing Philosophy*, 2011(12), 94–106.

Edmonson, C. (2010) 'Moral courage and the nurse leader', *The Online Journal of Issues in Nursing*, 15(3).

Epstein, E. and Delgado, S. (2010) 'Understanding and addressing moral distress', *The Online Journal of Issues in Nursing*, 15(3), 1–12.

Ferguson, Y. (2013) 'Critical reflection in statutory work', in J. Fook, J. and F. Gardner (Eds) *Critical Reflection in Context Applications in Health and Social Care* (London and New York: Routledge), pp. 83–92.

Field, J. (1983) *On Not Being Able to Paint* (Los Angeles: J.P. Tarcher Inc.).

Fleming, I. and Steen, L. (2011) *Supervision and Clinical Psychology: Theory, Practice and Perspectives*, 2nd edn (Hove: Routledge).

Fook, J. (2000) 'The lone crusader constructing enemies and allies in the workplace', in L. Napier, L. and J. Fook (Eds) *Breakthroughs in Practice Theorising Critical Moments in Social Work* (London: Whiting and Birch), pp. 186–200.

Fook, J. (2002) *Social Work Critical Theory and Practice* (London, Thousand Oaks and New Delhi: Sage).

Fook, J. (2010) 'Beyond reflective practice: reworking the "critical" in critical reflection', in H. Bradbury, N. Frost, S. Kilminster and M. Zukas (Eds) *Beyond Reflective Practice Approaches to Professional Lifelong Learning* (London: Routledge), pp. 37–51.

Fook, J. (2013) 'Critical reflection in context contemporary perspectives and issues', in J. Fook, and F. Gardner (2013) *Critical Reflection in Context Applications in Health and Social Care* (London and New York: Routledge), pp. 1–11.

Fook, J. and Askeland, G. (2006) 'The "critical" in critical reflection', in S. White, J. Fook and F. Gardner (Eds) *Critical Reflection in Health and Social Care* (Maidenhead: Open University Press), pp. 40–53.

Fook, J. and Gardner, F. (2007) *Practising Critical Reflection: A Resource Handbook* (Maidenhead: Open University Press).

Fook, J. and Gardner, F. (2013) *Critical Reflection in Context Applications in Health and Social Care* (London and New York: Routledge).

Fook, J., White, S. and Gardner, F. (2006) 'Critical reflection: a review of contemporary literature and understandings', in S. White, J. Fook and F. Gardner (Eds) *Critical Reflection and Professional Practice* (London: Open University Press), pp. 3–20.

Fowler, J.W. (1981) *Stages of Faith: The Psychology of Human Development and the Quest for Meaning* (San Francisco: Harper & Row).

Freshwater, D. (2002) 'Guided reflection in the context of post-modern practice', in C. Johns (Ed.) *Guided Reflection and Advancing Practice* (Oxford: Blackwell Publishing), pp. 225–38.

Freshwater, D. (2011a) 'Using reflection as a tool for research', in G. Rolfe, M. Jasper and D. Freshwater, *Critical Reflection in Practice Generating Knowledge for Care* (Houndmills: Palgrave Macmillan), pp. 183–95.

Freshwater, D. (2011b) 'Clinical supervision and reflection practice', in G. Rolfe, M. Jasper and D. Freshwater, *Critical Reflection in Practice Generating Knowledge for Care* (Houndmills: Palgrave Macmillan), pp. 100–26.

Freshwater, D. and Rolfe, G. (2001) 'A politically and ethically engaged method for nursing', *Nursing Times Research*, 6(1), 526–37.

Fronek. P., Kendall, M., Ungerer, G., Malt, A., Eugarde, E. and Geraghty, T. (2009) 'Towards healthy professional-service user relationships: The value of an interprofessional training course', *Journal of Interprofessional Care*, 23(1), 16–19.

Gaitskell, S. and Morley, M. (2008) 'Supervision in occupational therapy: how are we doing?', *The British Journal of Occupational Therapy*,71(3), 119–21.

Gardner, F. (2006) *Working with Human Service Organisations: Creating Connections for Practice* (Melbourne: Oxford University Press).

Gardner, F. (2007) 'Creating a climate for change', *International Journal of Knowledge, Culture and Change Management*, 6(7).

Gardner, F. (2011) *Critical Spirituality: A Holistic Approach to Contemporary Practice* (Farnham: Ashgate).

Gardner, F. (2012) 'The car, the rain and meaningful conversation: reflexivity and practice', in S. Witkin (Ed.) *The Call to Social Construction: Social Work as Relational Practice* (Columbia: Columbia University Press), pp. 103–26.

Gardner, F. (2013) 'Using critical reflection to research practice in a mental health setting', in J. Fook and F. Gardner (Eds) *Critical Reflection in Context Applications in Health and Social Care* (London and New York: Routledge), pp. 68–79.

Gardner, F. and Nolan, I. (2009) *Pastoral Care Networks Project* (Melbourne: Latrobe University).

Gardner, F. and Nunan, C. (2007) 'How to develop a research culture in a human services organisation: integrating research and practice with service and policy development' *Qualitative Social Work*, 6(3), 335–51.

Gardner, F., Rumbold, B. and Salau, S. (2009) *Strengthening Palliative Care in Victoria Through Health Promotion Project Report* (Melbourne: Palliative Care Unit, La Trobe University).

Gardner, F. and Taalman, E. (2013) 'Critical reflection and supervision: an interdisciplinary experience', in J. Fook and F. Gardner (Eds) *Critical Reflection in Context Applications in Health and Social Care* (London and New York: Routledge), pp. 93–104.

Geller, E. (2001) 'A reflective model of supervision in speech-language pathology: process and practice', *The Clinical Supervisor*, 20(2), 191–200.

Ghaye, T. (2005) *Developing the Reflective Healthcare Team* (Oxford: Blackwell Publishing).

Ghaye, T. and Lilyman, S. (2000) *Reflection: Principles and Practice for Healthcare Professionals* (Wiltshire: Mark Allen Publishing Ltd).

Giddens, A. (1999) *Runaway World How Globalisation is Reshaping Our Lives* (London: Profile Books).

Gould, N. (2004) 'The learning organization and reflective practice – the emergence of a concept', in N. Gould and M. Baldwin (Eds) *The Learning Organization and Reflective Practice–the Emergence of a Concept* (Aldershot, UK: Ashgate), pp. 1–9.

Grace, M. and Coventry, L. (2010) 'The co-location of YP4 and Centrelink in Bendigo', *Australian Journal of Social Work*, *10*, 157–74.

Grace, M., Coventry, L. and Battenham, D. (2012) 'The role of interorganization collaboration in "joined-up" case management', *Journal of Interprofessional Care*, 26(2) 141–9.

Guransky, D., Harvey, J. and Kennedy, R. (2003) *Case Management Policy, Practice and Professional Business* (Crows Nest, NSW: Allen & Unwin).

Gustafsson, G., Eriksson, S., Strandberg, G. and Norberg, A. (2010) 'Burnout and perceptions of conscience among health care personnel: A pilot study', *Nursing Ethics*, *17*(1), 23–38.

Hanlon, G. (2009) Unpublished reflective assignment, La Trobe University, Bendigo.

Harle, T., Page, M. and Ahmad, Y. (2010) 'Organizational issues', in K.C. Pollard, J. Thomas and M. Miers (Eds) *Understanding Interprofessional Working in Health and Social Care* (London: Palgrave Macmillan), pp. 138–55.

Hawkins, P. and Shohet, R. (2006) *Supervision in the Helping Professions*, 3rd edn. (Maidenhead: Open University Press McGraw Hill).

Healy, Karen. (2000) *Social Work Practices Contemporary Perspectives on Change* (London: Sage).

Hearne, B. (2013) 'Learning to play hide-and-seek with pink elephants', in J. Fook and F. Gardner (Eds) *Critical Reflection in Context Applications in Health and Social Care* (London and New York: Routledge), pp. 127–39).

Heelas, P. and Woodhead, L. (2005) *The Spiritual Revolution Why Religion is Giving Way to Spirituality* (Oxford: Blackwell Publishing).

Heron, J. and Reason, P. (1997) 'A participatory inquiry paradigm', *Qualitative Inquiry*, *3*(3), 274–94.

Hertz, R. (1997) (ed.) *Reflexivity and Voice* (Thousand Oaks, CA: Sage).

Hick, S.F. and Bien, T. (Eds) (2008) *Mindfulness and the Therapeutic Relationship* (New York/London: Guilford Press).

Hickson, H. (2011) 'Critical reflection: reflecting on learning to be reflective', *Reflective Practice*, *12*(6), 829–39.

Hickson, H. (2012) 'Reflective practice online: exploring the ways social workers used an online blog for reflection', *Journal of Technology in Human Services*, *30*(1), 32–48.

Hickson, H. (2013) 'Exploring how social workers learn and use reflection', unpublished PhD thesis, La Trobe University, Melbourne.

Holloway, M. and Moss, B. (2010) *Spirituality and Social Work* (Houndmills: Palgrave Macmillan).

Huffington, C., Armstrong, D., Halton, W., Hoyle, L. and Pooley, J. (2004) *Working Below the Surface. The Emotional Life of Contemporary Organizations* (London: Karnac).

Hughes, L. (1994) *The Collected Poems of Langston Hughes* (A. Rampersand and D. Roessel, Eds). (New York: Knopf).

Hughes, M. and Heycox, K. (2005) 'Promoting reflective practice with older people: learning and teaching strategies', *Australian Social Work*, *58*(4), 344–56.

Ife, J. (2008) *Human Rights and Social Work: Towards Rights Based Practice* (Port Melbourne: Cambridge University Press).

International Federation of Social Workers (n.d.) 'Statement of ethical principles', http://ifsw.org/policies/statement-of-ethical-principles/

Iversen, R.I., Gergen, K. and Fairbanks, R.P. (2005) 'Assessment and social construction: conflict or co-creation?', *British Journal of Social Work*, *35*, 689–708.

Jarvis, P. (2012) *Adult Education and Life Long Learning Theory and Practice* (Hoboken: Taylor and Francis).

Jasper, M. (2011) 'Understanding reflective writing', in G. Rolfe, M. Jasper and D. Freshwater (Eds) *Critical Reflection for Nursing and the Helping Professions Generating Knowledge for Care* (Houndmills: Palgrave Macmillan), pp. 52–73.

Jensen, G.M., Royeen, C. and Purtilo, R.B. (2010) 'Interprofessional ethics in rehabilitation: the dreamcatcher journey', *Journal of Allied Health*, *39*(3), 246–51.

Johns, C. (2005a) 'Balancing the winds', *Reflective Practice*, *6*(1), 67–84.

Johns, C. (2005b) 'Expanding the gates of perception', in C. Johns and D. Freshwater (Eds) *Transforming Nursing through Reflective Practice*, 2nd edn (Oxford: Blackwell), pp. 1–12.

Johns, C. and Freshwater, D. (2005) *Transforming Nursing through Reflective Practice*, 2nd edn (Oxford: Blackwell Publishing).

Johnson, R. (1986) *Inner Work* (San Francisco: Harper Row).

Johnson, R. (1993) *Owning Your Own Shadow* (San Francisco: Harper Row).

Jung, C.G. (1968) *The Archetypes and the Collective Unconscious*, 2nd edn, vol. 9, pt. 1 (Princeton, NJ: Princeton University Press).

Kadushin, A. (1985) *Supervision in Social Work* (New York: Columbia University Press).

Keddell, E. (2011) 'A constructionist approach to the use of arts-based materials in social work education: making connections between art and life', *Journal of Teaching in Social Work*, *31*(4), 400–14.

Keenan, M. (2012) 'Opening a space for hope in a landscape of despair: trauma and violence work with men who have sexually abused minors', in S. Witkin (ed.), *Social Construction and Social Work Practice* (New York: Columbia University Press), pp. 240–77.

Kolb, A. and Kolb, D. (2005) 'Learning styles and learning spaces: enhancing experiential learning in higher education', *Academy of Management Learning and Education*, *4*(2), 193–212.

Kumsa, M.K. (2012) 'When woman-at-risk meets youth-at-risk: engaging the discursive practices of the nation-state', in S.L. Witkin (ed.) *Social Construction and Social Work Practice* (New York: Columbia University Press), pp. 308–34.

Laabs, C. (2011) 'Perceptions of moral integrity: Contradictions in need of explanation', *Nursing Ethics*, *18*(3), 431–40.

Ladyshewsky, R. and Gardner, P. (2008) 'Peer assisted learning and blogging: a strategy to promote reflective practice during clinical fieldwork', *Australasian Journal of Educational Technology*, *24*(3), 241–57.

Lam, C.M., Wong, H. and Leung, T.T.F. (2007) 'An unfinished reflexive journey: social work students' reflection on their placement experiences', *British Journal of Social Work*, *37*, 91–105.

Lartey, E.Y. (2003) *In Living Color An Intercultural Approach to Pastoral Care and Counseling*, 2nd edn (London and Philadelphia: Jessica Kingsley).

Levine, D.M., Becker, D.M., Bone, L.R., Hill, M.N., Tuggle, M.B. and Zeger, S.L. (1994) 'Community-academic health center partnerships for underserved minority populations', *Journal American Medical Association*, *272*(4), 309–11.

Li, L.C., Grimshaw, J.M., Nielsen, C., Judd, M., Coyte, P.C. and Graham, I.D. (2009) 'Evolution of Wenger's concept of community of practice', *Implementation science*, *4*(11), 11–18.

Liddell, M. (2003) *Developing Human Service Organisations* (Frenchs Forest, NSW: Pearson SprintPrint).

Marks, D. (2008) 'Physical disability', in M. Davies (Ed.) *The Blackwell Companion to Social Work*, 3rd edn (Oxford: Blackwell), pp. 41–8.

Martin, S. (2009) 'Illness of the mind or illness of the spirit? Mental health-related conceptualization and practices of older Iranian immigrants', *Health and Social Work*, *34*(2), 117.

McEwen, K. (2011) *Building Resilience at Work* (Bowen Queensland: Australian Academic Press).

McLean, T. (2007) 'Interdisciplinary Practice', in J. Lishman (Ed.) *Handbook for Practice Learning in Social Work and Social Care* (London: Jessica Kingsley), pp. 322–43.

Mena, K.C. and Bailey, J.D. (2007) 'The effects of the supervisory working alliance on worker outcomes', *Journal of Social Service Research*, 34(1), 55–65.

Mezirow, J. (Ed.) (2000) *Learning as Transformation* (San Francisco: Jossey-Bass).

Mezirow, J. (2012) 'Learning to think like an adult', in E.W. Taylor and P. Cranton (Eds) *The Handbook of Transformative Learning Theory, Research and Practice* (San Francisco Jossey-Bass), pp. 73–95.

Miers, M. (2010) 'Learning the new ways of working', in K.C. Pollard, J. Thomas and M. Micrs (Eds) *Understanding Interprofessional Working in Health and Social Care* (Houndmills: Palgrave Macmillan), pp. 74–89.

Moodley, R., Gielen, U.P. and Wu, R. (Eds.) (2013) *Handbook of Counseling and Psychotherapy in an International Context* (New York and London: Routledge).

Morgan, A. (2000) *What is Narrative Therapy?* (Adelaide: Dulwich Centre Publications).

Morley, C. (2008) 'Teaching critical practice: resisting structural domination through critical reflection', *Social Work Education*, 27(4), 407–21.

Morley, C. (2012) 'How does critical reflection develop possibilities for emancipatory change? An example from an empirical research project', *British Journal of Social Work*, 42(8), 1513–32.

Murray, J.S. (2010) 'Moral courage in healthcare: acting ethically even in the presence of risks', *Online Journal of Issues in Nursing*, 15(3), ms 2.

Nangle, J. (2008) *Engaged Spirituality Faith Life in the Heart of the Empire* (Maryknoll, NY: Orbis Books).

Ni Raghallaigh, M. (2011) 'Religion in the lives of unaccompanied minors: an available and compelling coping resource', *British Journal of Social Work*, 41(3), 539–56.

Noble, C. and Irwin, J. (2009) 'Social work supervision: an exploration of the current challenges in a rapidly changing social, economic and political environment', *Journal of Social Work*, 9(3), 345–58.

Obholzer, A. and Miller, S. (2004) 'Leadership, followership, and facilitating the creative workplace', in C. Huffington, D. Armstrong, W. Halton, L. Hoyle and J. Pooley (Eds) *Working Below the Surface The Emotional Life of Contemporary Organizations* (London: Karnac), pp. 33–48.

Oelefson, N. (2012) *Developing Reflective Practice A Guide for Students and Practitioners of Health and Social Care* (Banbury, UK: Lantern Publishing).

Oliver, B. and Keeping, C. (2010) 'Individual and professional identity', in K.C. Pollard, J. Thomas, and M. Miers (Eds) *Understanding Interprofessional Working in Health and Social Care* (Houndmills: Palgrave Macmillan), pp. 90–104.

Oliver. B. and Pitt, B. (2005) 'Youth work', in G. Barrett, D. Sellman and J. Thomas (Eds) *Interprofessional Working in Health and Social Care Professional Perspectives* (Houndmills: Palgrave Macmillan), pp. 170–83.

Owens, P., Springwood, B. and Wilson, M. (2012) *Creative Ethical Practice in Counselling and Psychotherapy* (London: Sage).

Parton, N. (2007) 'Social work practice in an age of uncertainty', in S. L. Witkin and D. Saleeby (Eds) *Social Work Dialogue: Transforming the Canon in Inquiry, Practice and Education* (Alexandra, VA: CSWE Press), pp. 144–66.

Patel, N. (2011) 'Difference and power in supervision', in I. Fleming and L.S teen *Supervision and Clinical Psychology: Theory, Practice and Perspectives*, 2nd edn (Hove: Routledge), pp. 96–117.

Paterson, R. (2011) 'Can we mandate compassion?' *Hastings Center Report, 41*(2), 20–23.

Payne, M. (1997) *Modern Social Work Theory*, 2nd edn (London: Macmillan).

Pierson, J. (2002) *Tackling Social Exclusion* (London: Routledge).

Pollard, K. C., Thomas, J. and Miers, M. (Eds.) (2010) *Understanding Interprofessional Working in Health and Social Care* (Basingstoke: Palgrave Macmillan).

Proctor, B. (2008) *Group Supervision A Guide to Creative Practice*, 2nd edn (London: Sage).

Ray, M. D. (1998) 'Shared borders: achieving the goals of interdisciplinary patient care', *American Journal of Health-System Pharmacists, 53*(July 1), 1369–74.

Redmond, B. (2004) *Reflection in Action* (Aldershot, UK: Ashgate).

Reed, M. and Canning, N. (Eds) (2010) *Reflective Practice in the Early Years* (London: Sage).

Reynolds, M. and Vince, R. (2004) 'Organizing reflection: an introduction', in M. Reynolds and R. Vince (Eds) *Organizing Reflection* (Aldershot, UK: Ashgate), pp. 1–14.

Rolfe, G. (2000) *Research, Truth and Authority Postmodern Perspectives on Nursing* (Basingstoke: Macmillan).

Rolfe, G. (2011a) 'Knowledge and practice', in G. Rolfe, M. Jasper and D. Freshwater (Eds) *Critical Reflection in Practice Generating Knowledge for Care* (Basingstoke: Palgrave Macmillan), pp. 11–30.

Rolfe, G. (2011b) 'Reflection-in-Action', in G. Rolfe, M. Jasper and D. Freshwater (Eds) *Critical Reflection in Practice Generating Knowledge for Care* (Basingstoke: Palgrave Macmillan), pp. 160–82.

Rolfe, G., Jasper, M. and Freshwater, D. (2011) *Critical Reflection in Practice Generating Knowledge for Care* (Basingstoke: Palgrave Macmillan).

Rose, M. and Best, D. (2005) *Transforming Practice through Clinical Education, Professional Supervision, and Mentoring* (Edinburgh: Elsevier).

Rosenau, P. (1992) *Post-Modernism and the Social Sciences Insights, Inroads and Intrusions* (Princeton, NJ: Princeton University Press).

Ruch, G. (2005) 'Relationship-based practice and reflective practice: holistic approaches to contemporary child care social work', *Child and Family Social Work, 10*, 111–23.

Ruch, G. (2009) 'Identifying "the critical", in a relationship-based model of reflection', *European Journal of Social Work, 12*(3), 349–62.

Ruether, R. R. (2006) *Goddesses and the Divine Feminine: A Western Religious History* (Berkeley: University of California Press).

Rumbold, B. (2003) 'Caring for the spirit: lessons from working with the dying', *Medical Journal of Australia, 179*, S11–S13.

Saunders, C. (1990) *Hospice and Palliative Care: An Interdisciplinary Approach* (Seven Oaks, UK: Hodder and Stoughton).

Savaya, R., Gardner, F. and Stange, D. (2011) 'Stressful encounters with social work service users a descriptive account based on critical experiences', *Social Work*, 56(1), 63–71.

Sawn, E. and Bailey, A. (2004) 'Thinking with feeling: the emotions of reflection', in M. Reynolds, and R. Vince (Eds) *Organizing Reflection* (Aldershot, UK: Ashgate), pp. 105–25.

Schatzki, T. (2006) 'On organizations as they happen', *Organization Studies*, 27(12), 1863–73.

Scheeres, H., Solomon, N., Boud, D. and Rooney, D. (2010) 'When is it OK to learn at work? The learning work of organizational practices', *Journal of Workplace Learning*, 22(1), 13–26.

Schön, D.A. (1983) *The Reflective Practitioner: How Professionals Think in Action* (New York: Basic Books).

Scott, D. (1993) 'Inter-organization collaboration: why is it so difficult? Can we do it better?', *Children Australia*, 18(4), 4–9.

Scott, D. (2005) 'Inter-organizational collaboration in family-centred practice: a framework for analysis and action', *Australian Social Work*, 58(2), 132–41.

Sneed, R. A. (2010) *Representations of Homosexuality Black Liberation Theology and Cultural Criticism* (New York: Palgrave Macmillan).

Stanworth, R. (2002) 'Attention: A potential vehicle for spiritual care', *Journal of Palliative Care*, 18(3), 192–5.

Sturgeon, D. (2010) '"Have a nice day": consumerism, compassion and health care', *British Journal of Nursing*, 19(16), 1047–51.

Stedmon, J. and Dallos, R. (Eds) (2009) *Reflective Practice in Psychotherapy and Counselling* (Maidenhead: Open University Press).

Sullivan, W. (1995) *Work and Integrity: The Crisis and Promise of Professionalism in America* (New York: Harper Business).

Tacey, D. (2011) *Gods and Diseases* (Sydney: Harper Collins).

Tan, A. L., Wettasinghe, M., Tan, S.C. and Hasan, M. (2010) 'Reflection of teaching: A glimpse through the eyes of pre-service science teachers', Paper presented at the Curriculum, Technology & Transformation for an Unknown Future Conference, Sydney, pp. 1–12.

Thomas, J. (2005) 'Issues for the future', in G. Barrett, D. Sellman and J. Thomas *Interprofessional Working in Health and Social Care Professional Perspectives* (Houndmills: Palgrave Macmillan), pp. 187–99.

Thomson, G. (2013) 'Not beating around the bush: critical reflection in a rural community health service', in J. Fook and F. Gardner (Eds) *Critical Reflection in Context Applications in Health and Social Care* (London and New York: Routledge), pp. 68–79.

Thompson, S. and Thompson, N. (2008) *The Critically Reflective Practitioner* (Basingstoke: Palgrave Macmillan).

Titchen, A. and Higgs, J. (2001) 'Towards professional artistry and creativity in practice', in J. Higgs and A. Titchen (Eds) *Professional Practice in Health, Education and the Creative Arts* (Oxford: Blackwell Science), pp. 273–90.

Trelfa, J. (2005) 'Faith in reflective practice', *Reflective Practice*, 6(2), 205–12.

Vachon, B., Durand, M. and LeBlanc, J. (2010) 'Using reflective learning to improve the impact of continuing education in the context of work rehabilitation', *Advances in Health Sciences Education*, 15(3), 329–48.

Valani, C.E. (2009) 'Personal conscience and the Problem of Moral Certitude', *Nursing Clinics of North America*, 44(4), 407–14.

VanSant, S.S. (2003) *Wired for Conflict the Role of Personality in Resolving Differences* (Gainseville, FL: Center for Applications of Psychological Type).

Vince, R. (2001) 'Power and emotion in organizational learning', *Human Relations*, 54(10), 1325–51.

Vince, R. (2002) 'The politics of imagined stability: a psychodynamic understanding of change at Hyder plc.', *Human Relations*, 55(10), 1189–208.

Walsh, T. (2012) 'Shedding light on the expert witness role in child protection work: the value of social constructionism', in S. Witkin (Ed.), *Social Construction and Social Work Practice Interpretations and Innovations* (New York: Columbia University Press), pp. 188–210.

Webber, M. and Nathan, J. (2010 *Reflective Practice in Mental Health: Advanced Psychosocial Practice* (London: Jessica Kingsley).

Welsh, M.A. and Dehler, G.E. (2004) 'P(l)aying attention: communities of practice and organized reflection', in M. Reynolds and R. Vince (Eds) *Organizing Reflection* (Aldershot: Ashgate), pp. 14–28.

Wenger, E. (2000) 'Communities of practice and social learning systems', *Organization*, 7, 225–46.

White, G. (2006) *Talking about Spirituality in Health Care Practice* (London: Jessica Kingsley).

White, J. (2008) 'Family therapy', in M. Davies (Ed.) *The Blackwell Companion to Social Work* (Oxford: Blackwell), pp. 175–83.

White, S., Fook, J. and Gardner, F. (Eds) (2006) *Critical Reflection in Health and Social Care.* (Maidenhead: Open University Press).

Wilhelmsson, M., Pelling, S., Uhlin, L., Dahlgren, L.O., Faresjo, T. and Forslund, K. (2012) 'How to think about interprofessional competence: A metacognitive model', *Journal of Interprofessional Care*, 26(2), 85–91.

Wood, J. and Schuck, C. (2011) *Inspiring Creative Supervision* (London: Jessica Kingsley Publishers).

Wright, J. (2009) 'Reflective practice through a psychodynamic lens', in J. Stedmon and R. Dallos (Eds) *Reflective Practice in Psychotherapy and Counselling* (Maidenhead: Open University Press), pp. 56–72.

Wright, J. and Bolton, G. (2012) *Reflective Writing in Counselling and Psychotherapy* (London: Sage).

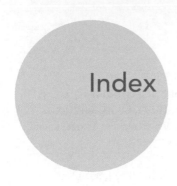

Index

Note: Page numbers in *italics* refer to figures.